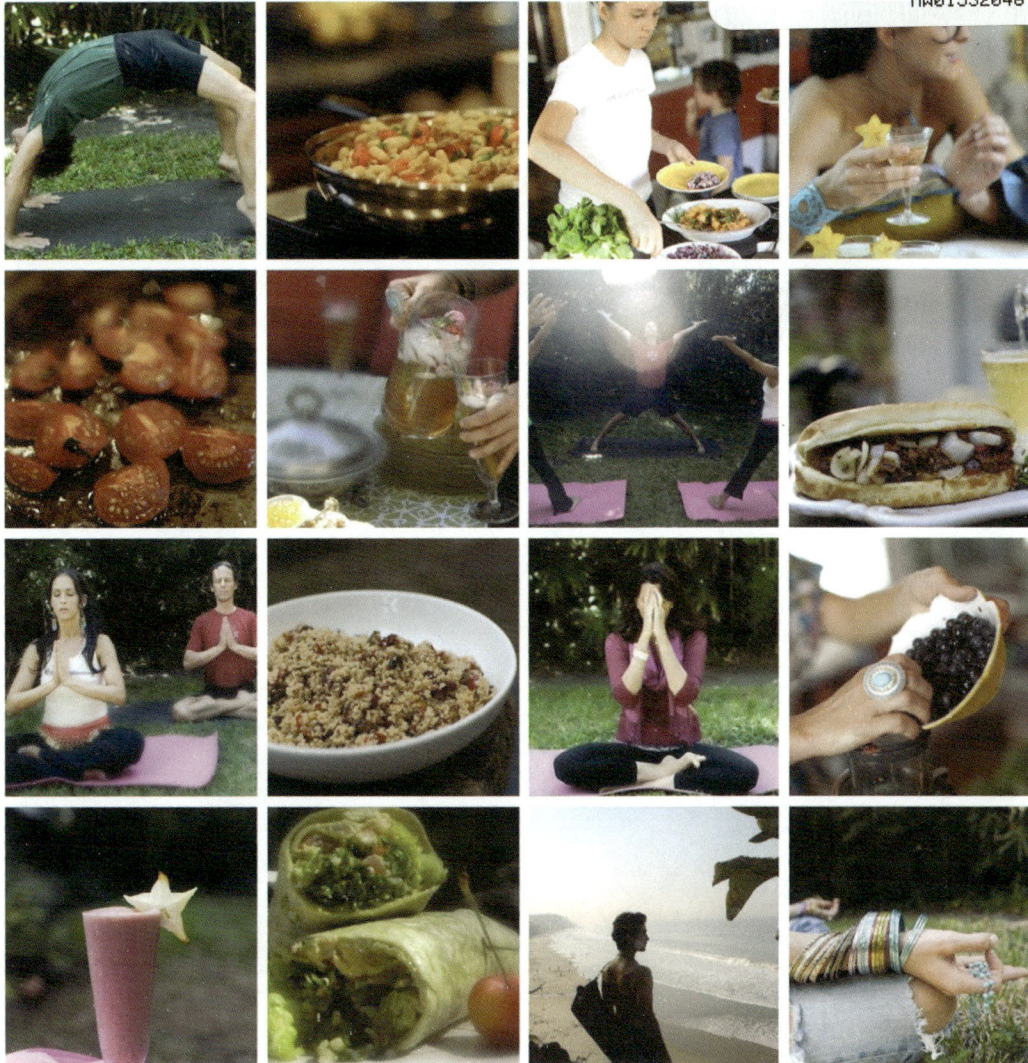

A PLANT-BASED, YOGIC LIFESTYLE INSPIRED BOOK

THE VEGAN MUSE & FRIENDS

A COLLECTION OF RECIPES & INSPIRATIONS FOR THE
PLANT-BASED, YOGIC LIFESTYLE

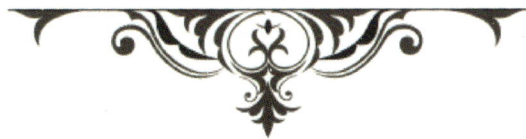

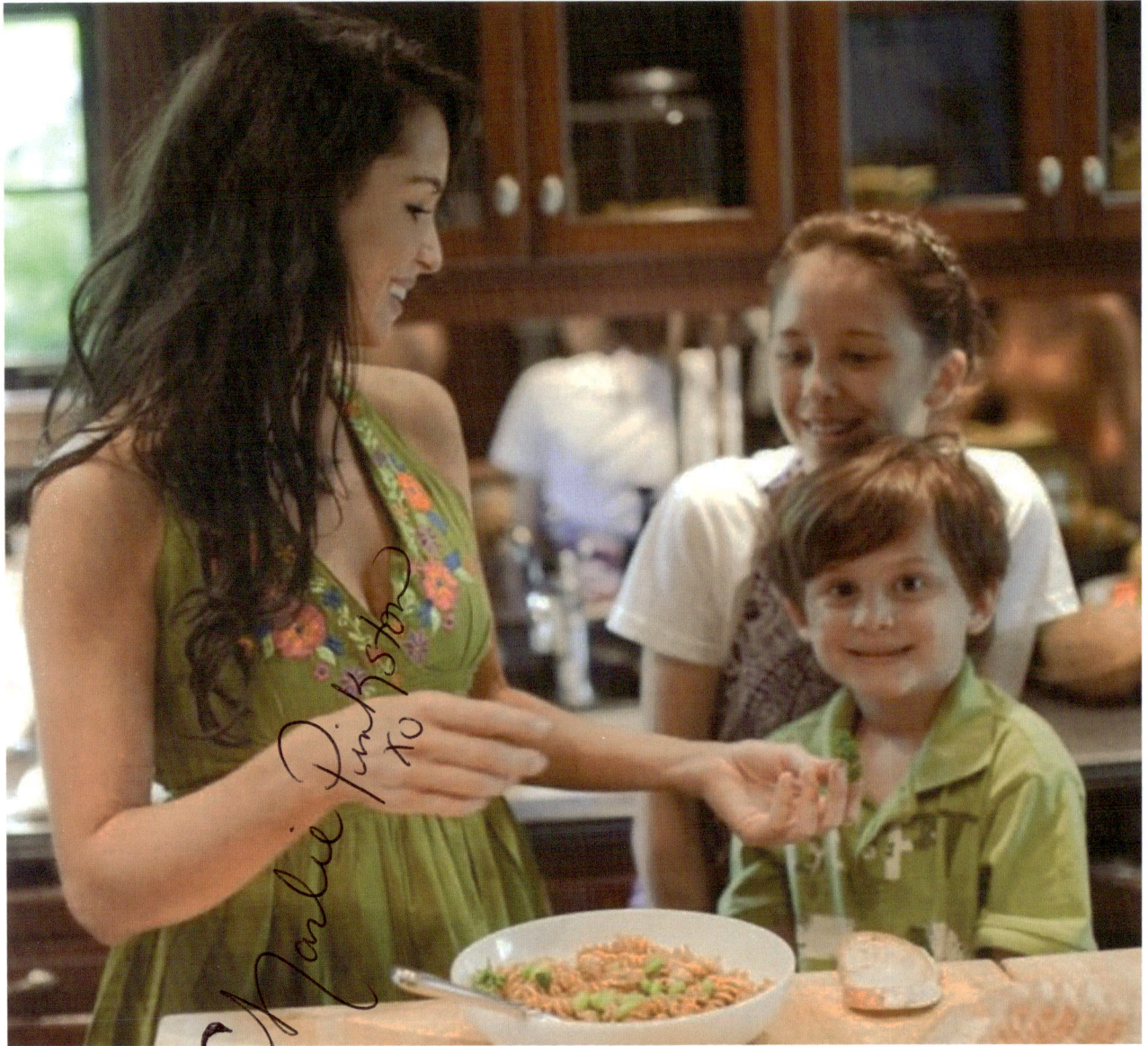

The kitchen is really is the soul of our home...I am never too far away from it and most of the time there is something simmering away for my family & friends. I am constantly thinking about ways to offer my inspirations on plant-based foods & yoga, the two make for a perfect courtship and have enhanced my life experience. I am overjoyed to be able to place a few of my favorite recipes, ideas, thoughts, inspirations & friends into this book for you to enjoy.

Welcome to our little corner of the world !

The Vegan Muse

& Friends

A collection of recipes & inspirations for the Vegan & Yogic Lifestyle

Charlie Pinkston

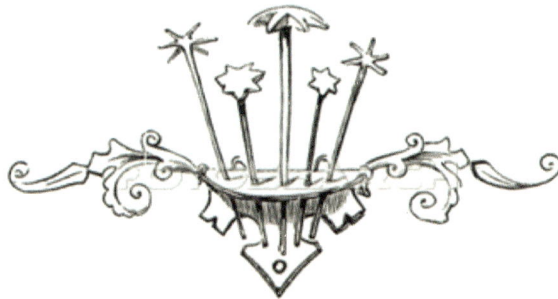

Photographs by Ruth Shepherd
& Charlie Pinkston

Edited By Kristen Ashton
& Renee Weaver

Author House Publisher

Lifestyle Book No.1
2011

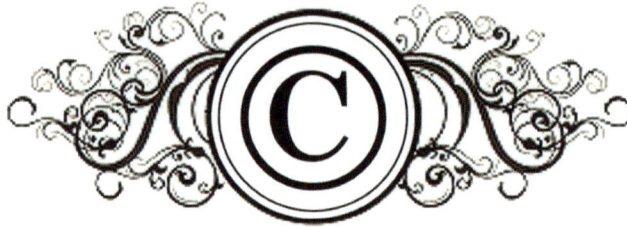

AuthorHouse™
1663 Liberty Drive
Bloomington, IN 47403
www.authorhouse.com
Phone: 1-800-839-8640

First published by AuthorHouse 3/17/2011

ISBN: 978-1-4567-5386-3 (sc)

Library of Congress Control Number: 2011903870

Printed in the United States of America

This book is printed on acid-free paper.

authorHOUSE®

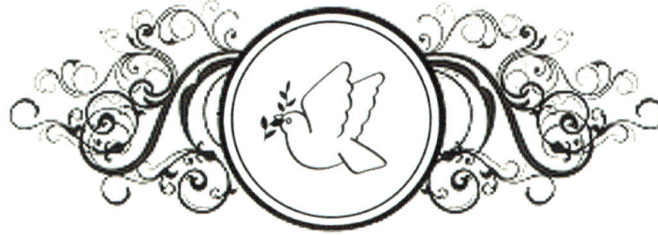

ACKNOWLEDGMENTS

To my lights: daughter, Madison and son, Jules. You make our house a home. You feed my soul like no other...and are my own personal muses in this life.

To my sister Renee: my best friend. Thank you for the long nights of moonlighting, for all of your work with this creation, and for speaking my language. Cheers to many more adventures.

To my teachers: Didier Razon and Ann Kiyonaga-Razon. It is an honor to have you both in my life. Thank you for offering yourselves each day to inspiring others with yoga.

To the featured friends of this book, foragers of goodness and light. You are world changers...you have embraced ethical lifestyles and have found ways to bring the message of compassion to others. Thank you for your contributions to this book.

Ong Namo Guru Dev Namo.

CONTENTS

FOREWORD

BY IAN M. KEOGH
CO-ORGANIZER
JACKSONVILLE'S RAW & LIVING FOODS GROUP

In November 1944, a visionary by the name of Donald Watson created the first newsletter for vegans aptly titled, "The Vegan News." Taking the first three letters and the last two letters from the title "vegetarian," Watson's goal for creating the term "vegan" was twofold. One, he wanted to designate a concise, positive term to reflect his group's mission to eliminate all animal products from one's diet. Watson understood that this may cause a split in the vegetarian movement, but he was quick to point out that both groups should be open to supporting each other's causes, and no animosity should exist among members of differently titled groups.

Watson's second goal, though, was a little more ambitious. "Should we adopt this," Watson wrote, "our diet will soon become known as a VEGAN diet, and we should aspire to the rank of VEGANS."[1] Watson was not content to merely have his newsletter become a hobby, but instead this "vegan" concept should be a movement, an ideal, and an identity that people should be reaching for! And, looking back at Watson's original newsletter, "vegan" has practically become a household name to describe this revolution in thinking, living, and eating.

Fast forward to the year 2010, and here enters another pioneering visionary by the name of Charlie Pinkston, The Vegan Muse. Inspired by this evolving lifestyle she has led since her teenage years, Charlie takes enormous amounts of pride in her plant-based creations, which have had a history of pleasing the senses and nourishing all of those around her. I have dubbed Charlie time and again "the vegan movement's best kept secret" with regards to her culinary talents, and a mere stroll through this book you hold in your hands confirms the reasons why.

In the spirit of Watson, Charlie recognizes the varying diet labels and lifestyles that encompass this movement, and wants to ensure support for any and all version of this "kind cuisine." And also in the spirit of Watson, our Muse has every intention to serve as a fountainhead of inspiration for all those who would like to follow her vision. She has done so many times over for me, already, and it is truly humbling to add a few words to this special book.

THE WORLD OF THE VEGAN MUSE NOW AWAITS
YOUR PARTICIPATION ...

1. Watson, D., "The Vegan News: Quarterly Magazine for the Non-Dairy Vegetarians", Vol. 1, No. 1, (November 24, 1944), p. 2.

IMPERATIVE INFORMATION

BY OLI DILLON SQUIRE
FEARLESS VEGAN, ANIMAL ACTIVIST AND CREATOR OF
WWW.ACTIONFOROURPLANET.COM

Much to my dismay, we live in a world full of cruelty, a world where animal exploitation is occurring on a tremendous scale. Chickens, for example, when battery farmed are shoved into tiny cages where they are unable to move. As a result, they begin to peck the other chickens to death because they are in such a mentally unhealthy environment. Many are de-beaked in an attempt to avoid cannibalism because of such close confinement with each other. The process of de-beaking causes chickens and turkeys agonizing pain. Male chicks are slaughtered at one day old because they are useless to the egg industry. Many will be thrown into a grinder, without receiving anesthetic, and will be ground alive. The plight of the pigs, cows, and other 'sweet' animals fair no better.

Imagine the human population of six to seven billion being culled around six times annually. It is a shocking thought nonetheless important in interpreting the sheer magnitude of slaughter. One can draw from these figures that animals are merely viewed as products to large corporations - cheap, indispensable products and nothing else. Unfortunately we live in a world where powerful companies are allowed to use deceptive tactics to fool consumers into buying a product. In many cases food companies label ingredients with a variety of long and complicated names instead of simply revealing the actual ingredients. One of the reasons they create these names is to disguise the shocking ingredients their foods contain. If the consumer knew what was in the food product they may think twice about buying it. Little do consumers know they may be consuming animal derivatives, animal collagen, animal tissue and animal hair. Many vegetarians and vegans may presume certain products do not contain any animal ingredients when, in fact, they do. It is very important for vegetarians and vegans to read and research all ingredients when purchasing foods and cosmetics as it is very easy to assume something will be animal free.

With all these facts exposed, it is incredibly surprising that the whole world is not vegetarian or at least more compassionate about animals. Simple steps such as cutting down on meat and eventually becoming vegetarian can make a big difference. Boycotting companies who sell fur and wearing faux fur alternatives, not buying products that have been tested on animals, and appreciating the beauty of nature can all make you a more caring consumer.

It is often difficult to get a precise figure of the number of species inhabiting our planet but scientists estimate that there are around three to thirty million species, two million of which are known. Such diversity compels one to pause for thought. With this diversity comes sheer beauty, magnificence and uniqueness. We are a privileged species being able to know of and admire the millions of wonderful other beings. Yet, from simply watching the news or reading the newspaper, it becomes confusing for compassionate beings to really understand why these creatures are becoming extinct and disregarded. Why do we humans feel it is acceptable to kill innocent animals for furs, food and products when we are intelligent enough to not do so?

Synthetic furs are available (often undistinguishable from real fur) and there are many varieties of meat free products out there. We have no need for oil from whales, the skin of cows and any other animal derived product. We are left questioning why we are doing this if the alternatives are out there and readily available. One argument is that humans are the dominant species and our ancestors have been eating animals since our species came into existence 200,000 years ago. It is drilled into our heads that this is a natural process and because it has been occurring for millennia it is deemed acceptable. However, being such an advanced species we need to realize the pain these animals suffer when being killed for meat, furs and products. Just like a human, they feel pain. Yet because they do not speak our language it seems to make it acceptable to mercilessly kill them, seeing as they can not respond and shout out in pain.

Vegetarians and vegans experience healthier lifestyles and have lower cholesterol as well as less chance of developing disease and illnesses. Vegetarians have around an extra seven years life span than those that constantly eat meat, as it is very unhealthy for the body.

With all these facts in mind, give being a vegetarian or vegan a go today. Treat yourself to a healthier body, a more compassionate nature and become more environmentally friendly. You alone can save hundreds of animals a year by not eating meat, wearing fur and refusing to purchase products using animal ingredients or products tested on animals.

Discover the many reasons people are vegan…and see how you can make a difference.

ACTION FOR OUR PLANET WILL FEATURE A CAMPAIGN PAGE WITH INFORMATION ON THE ORGANIZATIONS INVOLVED, LINKS TO THEIR PETITIONS AND TO THE LATEST NEWS UPDATES.

~ BE INSPIRED…GET INVOLVED…MAKE A DIFFERENCE!

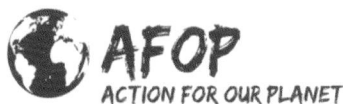

AFOP
ACTION FOR OUR PLANET

INTRODUCTION

We have all heard the titles: vegetarian, vegan, raw, raw-vegan, sustainable, slow, local, and organic. But, the thing is, we've heard these words so much our eyes have glazed over! To lighten the mood a bit, this book was created as my ode to plant-based lifestyle aficionados. I decided to add some special touches to the menu: simply, simple food made with whole grains, cleaner proteins (no faux meats), inspired tips, basic vegan recipes with a flare, raw juices for cellular cleansing, yoga, and of course, lots of mused inspirations -- a lovely combination for the mind, body, and soul.

This book's purpose is to bring you recipes to enchant your taste buds, entice your senses, and make you want to indulge in the divine goodness of healthy dishes. Eating well, focusing on the positive, and lifting your spirits while nurturing your soul are the greatest ingredients you can give yourself. You will only need a few things for this to take place: an appetite for change, an appetite for healthy, compassionate food, and an appetite for inspired focus.

I am now a firm believer that a plant-based diet, rich in whole grains, cleaner proteins, and fresh local fruits and vegetables is the healthiest plant-based diet. Although I do make the faux meats from time to time and am happy to have them available, they do not fit into my daily eating plans due to the highly processed ingredients.

These days, with my focus on nutrient-rich comfort foods, I have found my bliss. So, I hope to be a muse of sorts to you, a non-judgmental friend who vows to encourage, inspire, and entice you with recipes that will cultivate a newfound pleasure in eating and living a plant-based, yogic lifestyle.

My advice to you now is to take it slow if need be. Change can be difficult. Begin by adopting into your life a few days a week a healthy vegan diet. Find a health counselor for extra guidance and advice. Visit your local health food stores such as Grassroots Natural Market, Native Sun Natural Foods Market, Whole Foods Market, and Mother Earth (these are just some in my neck of the woods). These places will have a host of experts to assist you.

Remain faithful to your local farmers, as being a contributor to your community is the best way to go, always. Be a locavore and visit your Farmers' Markets to meet your local organic farmers; they will also be a great source of information for you. Be curious, sample fresh organic foods straight from Mother earth.

Fall in love with nature's exquisite bounty of nutrient-rich, body healing goodness all over again or for the first time. Take kale, for instance. This sweet, earthy bouquet of vibrantly rich greens holds not only great texture but an added layer of completeness to your dishes. The magical green, as I call it, is loaded with anti-cancer compounds called sulforaphanes as well as vitamins A, B, and C. Seek out blemish-free, dark-greens the next time you visit your local market or farm stand.

A question that often arises is about vitamin B-12...Do plant-based folks get enough? There are many ways to obtain the adequate amounts...one way to is to simply incorporate some nutritional yeast into your diet. The mere amount of B-12 needed per day is about 2.5 micro grams. Drinking fortified rice or soy milk is another instant dose of this required vitamin. To simply sum up a vegan diet: it is a generous supply of legumes, nuts, whole grains, fruits, and vegetables that provide a plethora of vital nutrients as well as protection against diseases such as cardiovascular disease, cancer, and so many more.

As seekers of a more enlightened diet, be aware of being misled by the overused "organic label" of many companies. By making your produce purchases from your local farms, not only are you controlling your choice of food intake, but you are also helping to eliminate the thousands of air miles used to bring in outside products to the local chain stores. Be inspired to cultivate your own garden no matter how small; see the magic of a seed turned into a divine ingredient. Organic farming and gardening is respectful to our planet and the laws of nature.

Branch out and join groups to meet other like-minded folks; it is always important to have support nearby. Find a passion to learn more each day about the benefits food, yoga, juicing, and meditation have. By incorporating a few of these things into your lifestyle you will begin to feel your mind calmed, your body nourished, your spirit awakened, and your soul soothed. With so much divine goodness and newly found knowledge, we must be inspired to share the light with friends and family. These will truly be the first steps into your many compassionate culinary adventures.

There is a large amount of literature that suggests the consumption of a proper plant-based diet along with daily yoga is associated with lower blood pressure, lower cholesterol levels, less risk of heart disease, stroke, cancer, overall stability with emotions and healthier mental outlook on life. This knowledge, as well as my inner intuition, gives me the understanding that there is an amazing courtship that yoga and food have on our daily lives. Many who embrace the yogic lifestyle are taking on the plant-based diet. After practicing yoga and learning about ahimsa, meat looses its appeal... something just seems to click. This awareness, this found understanding of the lack of compassion that goes into what ends up on your plate is growing in vast numbers each day. As this awakening grows and the non-dual way of viewing things grows, a calm connectedness is felt.

Compassionate cuisine becomes a way of life. Compassion is the magic word that joins every being in the universe together. Through meditation and yoga, self awareness is reached because your mind-set begins to shift, your heart opens and compassion enters. With the understanding all universal life is connected and what we do affects all therein, we must consider how we treat all living creatures. Yoga is freedom. Confinement and suffering is slavery. One of the quotes of PETA says, "think before you eat." Although it is a simple quote, the message resonates on a deeper level. Once you begin to open your third eye (so to speak) and realize how the food on your plate came to be there, eating a creature that has endured slavery in the most inhumane ways, I believe, must be eliminated from your diet in order to truly free yourself and begin living from your heart.

Whether you desire a healthier approach to eating, want to lighten your environmental footprint, or you want to apply the principals of ahimsa, you must make certain you are obtaining enough key nutrients such as calcium, iron, B-12, and protein. Balancing meals with a variety of whole grains, organic veggies, fruits, and lean protein (such as beans and tofu) as well as healthy fats like avocados and nuts is a must if you are seeking a proper vegan diet. Eliminating the animal from one's diet can seem overwhelming; very few people become entirely vegan overnight. It is a gradual process but can become a reality if one is motivated to learn more about the benefits of the plant-based lifestyle.

This courtship of yoga and food inspires me to a place of balance, a place where I feel completely at peace ~ both inside myself and out.

Cheers to blissfully balanced, new awakenings
Charlie

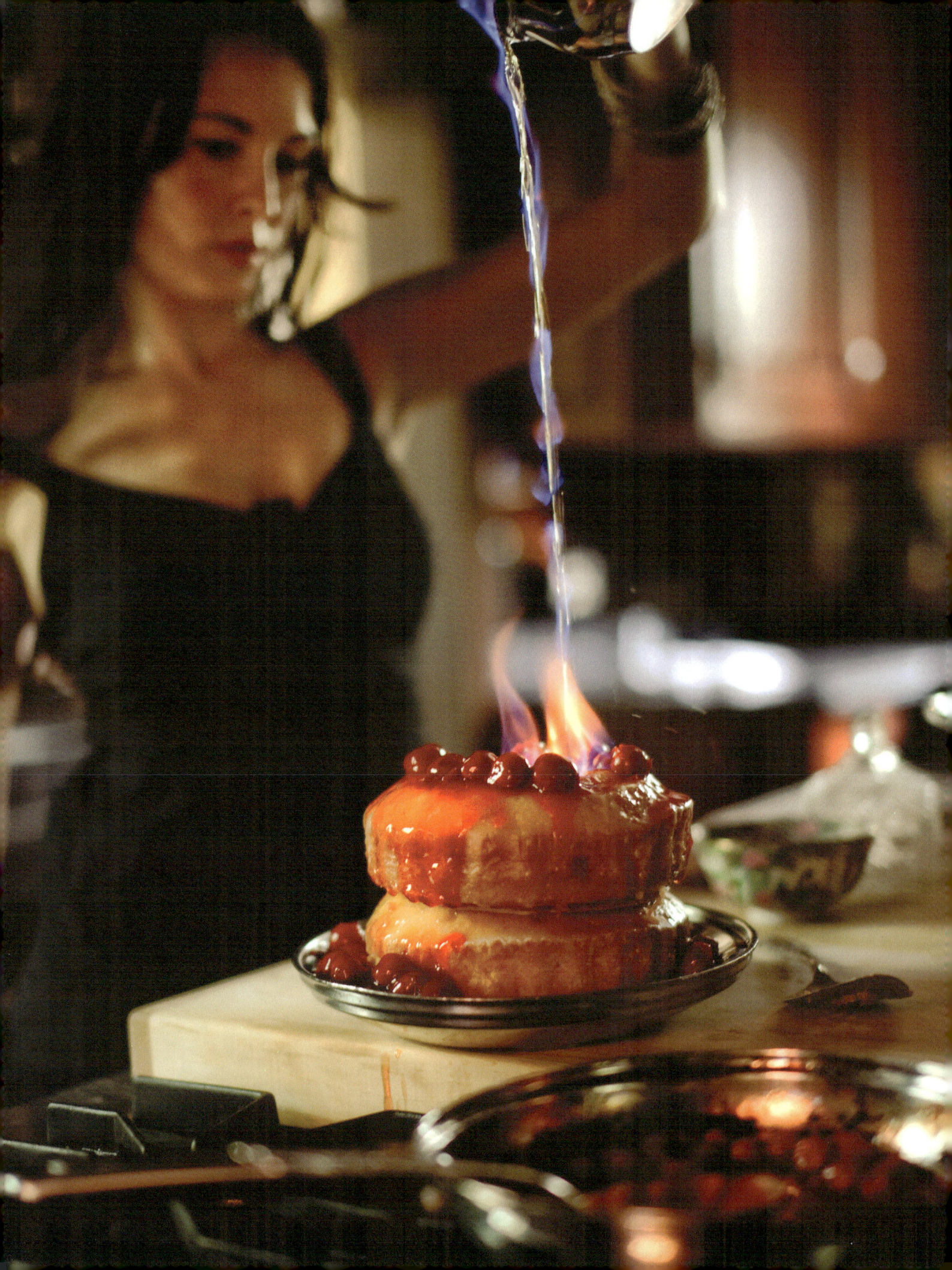

KITCHEN & PANTRY MUSINGS

By simply replacing your white flours, refined sugars, and unhealthy oils with whole grain flours, natural raw sugars, and healthy oils, you will feel the difference in your overall well-being. You will increase your chances of experiencing an awakening and empowering feeling, a magical sensation for your mind, body, and soul. Remember, the goal is to eliminate the negative and accentuate the positive.

If you have to start small by purchasing a few staples and build as you go, your pantry stash will begin growing into a healthy oasis in due time. To keep things simplistic, I am only listing what I like to keep in my own pantry…you will have fun finding your own personal favorites. These favorites will create a path and a simple foundation by which you can begin cultivating your way into dining on compassionate cuisine as well as keeping the costs of living down. I have heard so many people tell me that going vegan seems like it would be too expensive. My response is that I keep our dishes simple, seasonal, local, and creative using products that induce instant doses of health and provide layers of flavorful ingredients. Whole grain rice and protein rich beans are an inexpensive foundation in which to begin with when concocting meal plans. Another bonus is that by eliminating known cancer causing meats and allergen enhancing dairy products from our diet, this keeps the number of doctor's visits down. Staying out of the doctor's office is truly a less expensive way of living!

From the plant world, you can get all the calcium that you need. Some good sources are beans, leafy greens, almonds, and broccoli. If there is a concern for iron, no worries. You can find numerous ways to obtain your needed amount from nuts, whole grains, leafy greens, beans, and a plethora of other vegetables. Numerous studies show eggs, cheeses, and dairy are the cause for our most dreaded diseases. The elimination of these foods is not only ethical but healthy. If you still desire these types of foods, I have placed a few alternatives for you to explore. Please be mindful to read labels and understand the ingredients with all foods that are not whole. Also, remain consciously aware of the amount of faux products you consume, as it is most beneficial to remain as clean with your diet as possible

Musing No. 1

Create a pantry boudoir. Treat your staples just as you would your best designer baubles and garments. Arrange, organize, showcase, and display your glorious goodies!

THE TRANSITIONS

HERE ARE SOME PRODUCT SUGGESTIONS TO EASE YOURSELF INTO THE ELIMINATION OF EGGS, DAIRY, AND MEAT.

Cream Cheese - Tofutti's Better Than Cream Cheese
Sour Cream - Tofutti - Better than Sour Cream, non-hydrogenated
Ice Cream - Luna & Larry's Coconut Bliss
Eggs - Ener-G Egg Replacer
Cheddar Cheese Shreds - Daiya, Cheddar Style Shreds
Sausage - Lightlife, Gimme Lean Ground Sausage or Tofurky, Italian Sausage
Bacon - Lightlife, Smart Bacon
Pizza - Tofurky, Pepperoni or Cheese Pizzas
Deli Slices - Tofurky, Hickory Smoked, Oven Roasted, and Peppered
Pepperoni - Tofurky, Pepperoni Deli Slices
Turkey - Tofurky Roast
Mayo - Vegenaise
Butter - Earth Balance, Organic Buttery Spread
Milks - Coconut, Hemp, Soy, Almond, Oat and Rice milks are very popular.

THE FRESH

ITS ALWAYS A GOOD IDEA TO KEEP FRESH PRODUCE STOCKED...GOOD FOR SOUPS, JUICING ROUTINES, AND SNACKS. LETTING GO OF THE OVERLY PROCESSED, OR NON-ORGANIC PRODUCE, AND FOODS WILL BE ONE OF THE BEST THINGS YOU CAN OFFER YOURSELF AND YOUR LOVED ONES.

Kale, Chard, Bok Choy, Napa Cabbage, Carrots, Onions, Broccoli, Leeks, Cucumbers, Apples, Celery, Pears, Lemons, Parsley, Mint, Cilantro, Basil, Rosemary, Sage, Thyme, Tarragon, Garlic, Ginger…these are just a few of my favorites. Find your favorites to keep on hand.

THE PANTRY

This section is merely a basic starting point towards your goals of healthful ingredients such as whole grains, whole grain flours, minimally processed meat replacements, oils, natural sweeteners, etc. Expand your pantry mindset. Infuse your kitchen with doses of conscious changes. When you begin setting up your stock, do not become overwhelmed with replacing the old with the new straight away. Take it step by step and allow it to evolve. Recipes in this book, by design, were formulated to use many of the same ingredients. As this is a way to limit cost and have an over all stress free way to begin or improve your current vegan journey. Having shelves full of esoteric ingredients to make your dishes delicious, I feel, is NOT needed. One secret I must divulge is I ritualistically keep an uncomplicated approach to making my dishes. Focus instead on the layers, textures, and overall companionship of the flavors used. I'd rather light some candles, pour a smidgen of wine, turn on some music, get into my zen place, and cook than to spend a whole day shopping for ingredients I may only use once or twice.

WHOLE GRAINS
Brown Rice, Wild Rice, Brown Basmati, Barley, Quinoa, Oats

SWEETS FOR THE SWEET
Agave Nectar, Brown Rice Syrup, Pure Maple Syrup, Blackstrap Molasses, Turbinado, Vegan Dark Chocolate

OILS
Extra Virgin Olive Oil First Cold Pressed, Extra Virgin Coconut Oil (I like the Garden of Life brand), Flaxseed Oil, Sesame Oil, Safflower Oil

FLOURS
Oat Flour, Whole Wheat Pastry, White Whole Wheat Pastry, Spelt Flour

FERMENTED MUST HAVES
Un-pasteurized Naturally Fermented Miso Paste, Balsamic Vinegar, Shoyu, Bragg's Apple Cider Vinegar, Bragg's Liquid Aminos, Ume Plum Vinegar, Tarragon Vinegar, Brown Rice Vinegar, Umeboshi Vinegar, Mirin

BEANS
Black, Red, Pink, Kidney, Pinto, and White Beans, Chickpeas, Lentils, Black-Eyed Peas, Edamame (freshly shelled)

SEA VEGGIES
Nori, Hijiki, Wakame, Arame, Agar-Agar

HERBS, SPICES, & WHAT-NOT'S
Paprika, Turmeric, Curry, Chili Pepper, Cumin, Oregano, Sage, Rosemary, Thyme, Fennel, Coriander, Dill, Basil, Ginger, Garlic, Sea Salt, Ground Pepper, Cinnamon, Nutmeg, Cloves, Pure Vanilla Extract, Pure Almond Extract

SEEDS & NUTS
Sesame Seeds, Pumpkin Seeds, Flax Seeds, Sunflower seeds, Almonds, Pine Nuts, Walnuts, Pecans, Tahini, Nut Butters

FRUITS
Fresh seasonal fruit is best if possible - Dried Fruits, Raisins, Pineapple, Apricots, Dates, Cranberries, Figs

PASTAS
Whole Wheat, Rice Noodles, Soba Noodles

MY FAVORITE QUICK CLEANSE
RAW Cleanse from Garden of Life, an easy-to-use, triple detox formula that eliminates toxins from the body in only one week.

MISCELLANEOUS
Trail Mix, Whole Grain Cereals (I like Ezekiel brand), Popcorn, Organic Fruit Spreads, Whole Wheat Tortillas, Sourdough Bread, Whole Grain Sourdough Bread, Yerba Maté, Matcha, Organic Vegetable Broth

KEY INGREDIENT & NUTRITION BANTER

It's all about expanding and embracing the idea of change - changes that will truly enrich our meals in more ways than one. Change is healthy and is a mantra worth surrendering to time and time again. I encourage you to look into your cupboards and begin to mindfully update your flours, rice, pasta, oils, sweeteners, ferments, herbs, and spices repertoire.

Using key ingredients like whole wheat, quinoa, and brown rice (just to list a few) are more healthful than the over used refined-flour versions. Whole grains are rich in fiber and a perfect ingredient to use in the reducing of heart disease amongst other health issues. Not only are they full of B vitamins, selenium, phytochemicals, and magnesium, but they are also gluten-free.

Quinoa, quinoa, quinoa…I am smitten by this "mother grain", (FYI…quinoa is a "pseudo grain", it is actually closely related to beets and spinach!) which was what the Incas called this wonder food. Unlike numerous other whole grains, this one in particular can be made on the fly as it only takes about 20 minutes to cook. It is one of the few complete sources of vegan proteins. It has all nine amino acids that are essential for building proteins in the body. Buying this in bulk is a "smarty-pants" move for a vegan as you can use it for breakfast, lunch, and dinner. On a crisp, cool morning, a bowl of quinoa porridge not only comforts the soul but also boosts your energy level.

A true culinary treasure to me is oils. The way the oils bring our dishes, sauces, and dressings to life is well worth stocking our pantry with healthier versions. Let go of certain ones such as canola and corn oil, as these tend to always be highly refined and produced with genetically modified corn. Gravitate toward coconut, almond, flax seed, and olive oil. It is surely quintessential bliss to adorn your dishes with natural and necessary saturated fats as opposed to the oils that are highly refined and have become damaged goods in the process of being created. Become an alchemist in your kitchen. Be inspired by the tropical and rich fragrance of the coconut oil, the earthy golden shade and rich in omega-3 acids of flax seed oil, and the rich in omega-9 fatty acids of the much used in our home, olive oil.

If you are relying on artificial sweeteners, know they have questionable ingredients that are linked to many diseases. Do your research! Your body is your temple; fill your temple with the goodness that is merely a market away. Avoid high-fructose corn syrup as this is one of the most used sweeteners in the U.S. It is found in sodas, processed foods, and a very long list of "convenient" foods. Not only has this been derived from genetically modified corn crops, but it has also gone through such an intense process chemically it has no resemblance whatsoever to the original crop.

We all at one point in time have used, or still do, white granulated sugar. This is not the glittery, enchanting fairy dust it looks like! Its pure sweetness was stripped of any character and flavor it once had. Unless your sugar is labeled "pure cane sugar," it is likely that you are consuming a highly processed and mostly pure sucrose product. My attainable fantasy sugar is the amber hued crystals of turbinado. Natural, raw, unbleached, unrefined, and fair trade certified are some of the magic words of this incredibly elegant treasure.

Many fermented foods help maintain your digestive tract and maintain a rather good partnership with the friendly bacteria in your body. Fermented staples have ways to delight the senses, add personality to your dishes, and evoke an influence of health on your intestinal flora. This enchanted culinary elixir comes in many forms. Vinegars, shoyu, and miso are some of my favorites. The way that apple cider vinegar can create a concoction of straight nutrition as well as lift the flavor of many dishes to an otherworldly level is just a small part of why this product is used so often in our home. Organic, un-pasteurized shoyu adds a layer of complexity and depth to almost any food. The chemically processed soy sauce is easy to toss out after the use of shoyu. Miso, the fermented soybean paste, has been a familiar ingredient to me for the past couple of years. The many uses of miso go beyond soup. Although I must say, The Shaman's Soup encompasses my love of miso and its plethora of healing powers.

Herbs and spices add healing properties that lend medicinal qualities. Herbs, spices, and seasonings are key to unlocking the balance of flavors desired for your dishes. Paring these fragrant, flavorful powders, salts, peppers, and herbs can create a poetic spectrum of culinary wonder. I gravitate towards the nostalgic sea salts for their trace minerals and clean flavor. They range in colors from rose quartz pink and obsidian black to the familiar white crystal. Explore the many varieties of pepper available such as tell cherry or pink and white peppercorns.

In Ayurveda, black pepper is known as a brain tonic, and who doesn't need one of those? Some of my favorite herbs and seasonings are garlic, turmeric, curry, ginger, rosemary, and basil. What are your favorites? Evaluate your stash and consider these layers of flavors and textures lacing your dishes to be one of the best tools in your kitchen. Since the dawn of humanity, herbs, spices, and seasonings were used as a form of currency. Their value brought about prolific conversations over the dinning table where I believe that the famous saying, "spice for conversation" just may have been cultivated!

Obtaining the vitamins and minerals needed each day is also not as hard as it may seem. For instance, iron can be found in nuts, enriched grains, and legumes. Sea veggies such as kelp, nori, and agar-agar are a quick way to obtain iodine. Leafy greens, figs, fortified non-dairy milks, tofu, and broccoli are packed with calcium. Creating a daily ritual of soaking up some sun rays will allow your body to absorb vitamin D. I hope that some of these brief suggestions will resonate with you and encourage you on a path of a well balanced plant-based lifestyle. So, grab some sea veggies, figs, and whirl a yummy leafy green salad together and head to the great outdoors for your quick dose of some vitamins today!

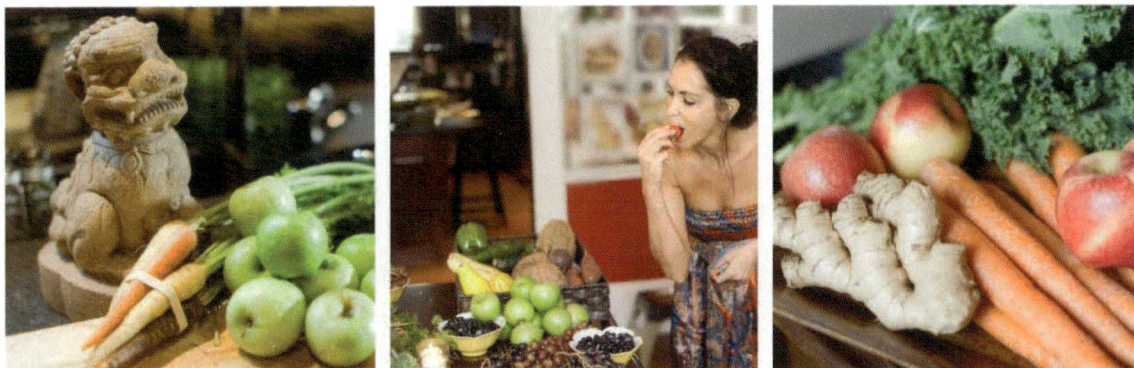

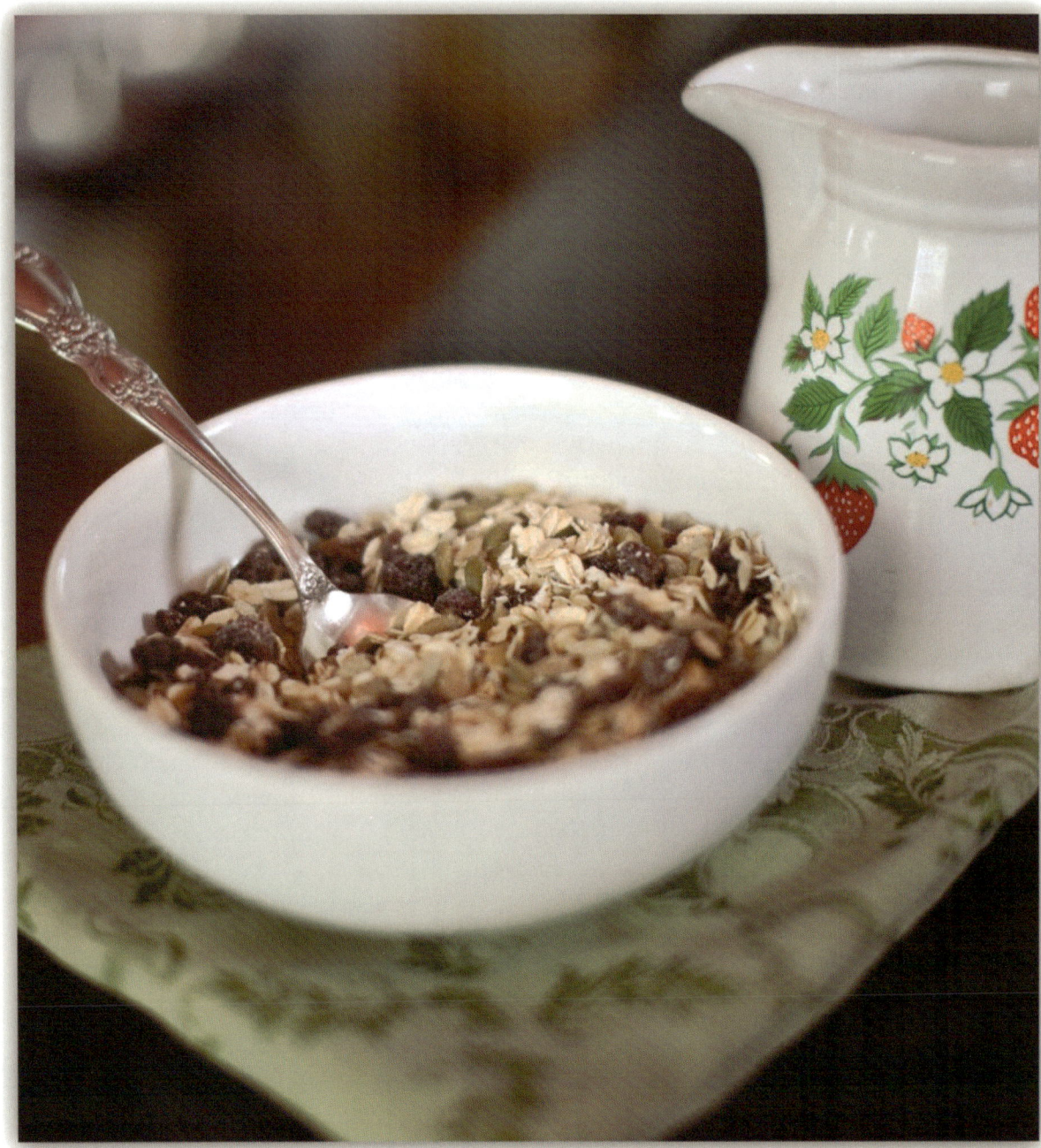

Musing No. 2

Whole grains will be one of the key factors of living the charmed, healthy, and well balanced plant-based lifestyle.

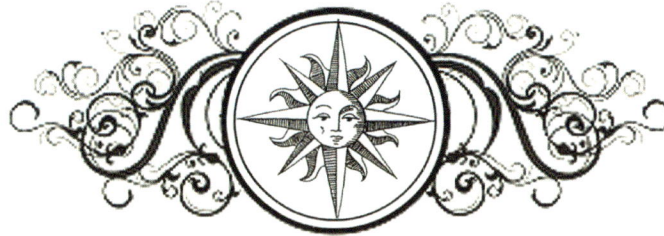

BREAKFAST

Be mindful and intuitive; sometimes the body only craves the simplest of things. Sipping your breakfast can be a quick way to get an instant dose of rich vitamins. With all of the colors that Mother Earth provides us in fruit and veggies, it's one way we can taste the rainbow of health and indulge in all that our bodies need. Begin this section by focusing your intentions on simple, spirit-lifting, and body nourishing ways to begin your days.

BANANA SCENTED PANCAKES

serves 4

You really can't go wrong with this one. It is one of my family's Sunday morning rituals. It's easy enough for my little ones to get in the kitchen and start the process. Of course, the shapes you make are up to you. My son, Jules, prefers a star shape while my daughter, Madison, loves to create the peace symbol with her batter. The experience of joining together as a family is very important to me. What are your weekend rituals? Make them fun, and keep them healthy for your family. Experiment with mixing in different nuts, seeds, and fruits for extra layers of flavor.

1 cup white whole wheat flour
½ tablespoon turbinado sugar
1 teaspoon baking powder, aluminum free
¼ teaspoon baking soda
¼ teaspoon sea salt
1 banana, mashed
1 ¼ cup almond milk
2 tablespoons coconut oil
pure maple syrup, for serving
Walnuts, for sprinkling

In a large bowl combine the flour, sugar, baking powder, baking soda, and salt. In a smaller bowl, mash the banana and add in 1 cup of milk and oil; mix together. If you find your batter to need a bit more milk - slowly add in a little at time. Create a well in the center of the flour mixture, and pour the wet mixture into the well. Lightly blend ingredients together until lumps are gone.

Heat skillet over high heat; make sure that your skillet has been heavily oiled (I use coconut oil for this).

Drop about ¼ cup of batter onto the hot skillet and allow to cook until the edges of cakes begin to lift and bubbles begin to appear on the top of the uncooked side. Flip and cook other side. Serve up with pure maple syrup and your favorite toppings. We like to sauté walnuts and bananas in the leftover coconut oil to top ours off.

Musing No. 3
Eat breakfast in bed more often.

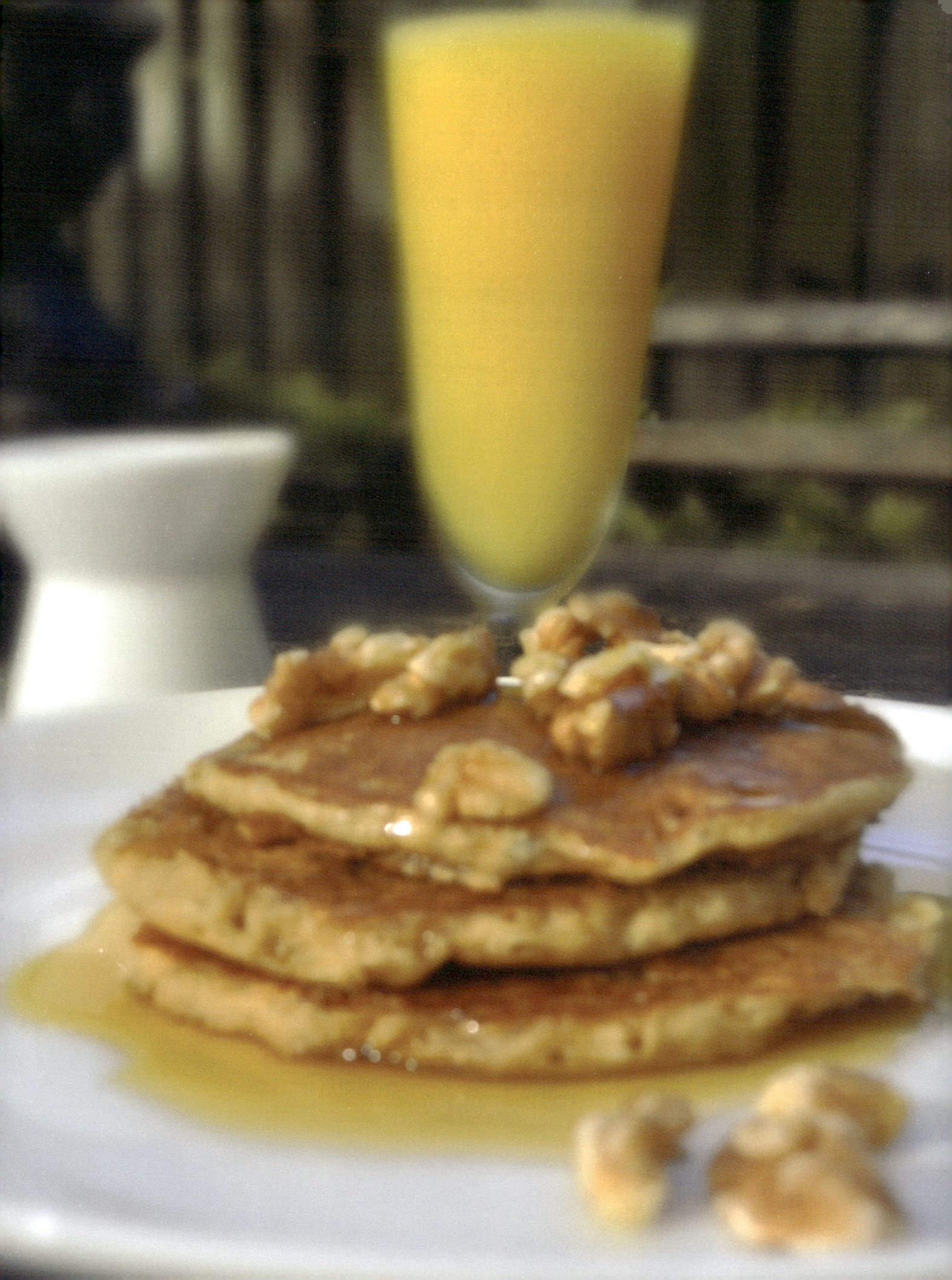

A GRAND HASH

serves 2 - 4

In our home, we use the expression, "The imperfections of life are half the charm." This is our positive mantra that we say to make light of the many bumps or lessons learned from life! For whatever reason, when something seems a bit off kilter, I am drawn to comfort foods. Sound familiar? When I say comfort foods, I do not mean heavy, junky foods. I mean those foods that have a nostalgic flavor, the foods that create a waft of deliciousness in your home.

4 medium potatoes, diced
3 tablespoons extra virgin olive oil
½ cup scallions, chopped
1 package tempeh, cut into ½ inch cubes
2 ½ tablespoons shoyu
½ tablespoon garlic, minced
¼ teaspoon paprika
¼ cup fresh parsley, chopped
sea salt and fresh ground pepper
to taste

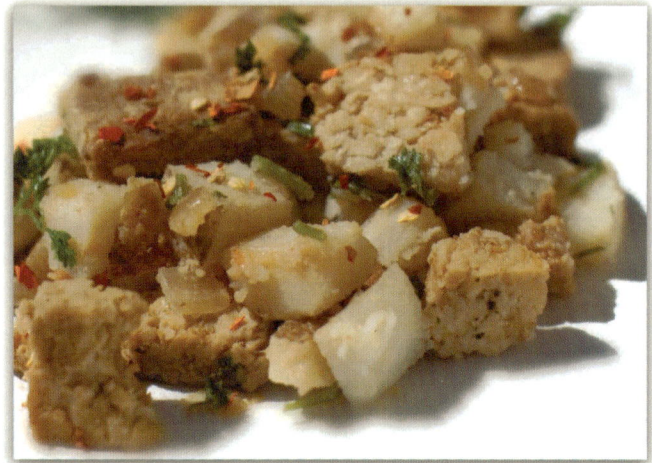

Cover potatoes with water in a large pot. Sprinkle in a bit of sea salt and bring water to a boil. Allow to cook for 10 - 15 minutes or until tender. Drain.

In a large skillet drizzled with olive oil, sauté the scallions, tempeh, and shoyu, stirring frequently to cook all sides of tempeh. Add in garlic, paprika, parsley, salt, pepper, and potatoes. Mix well.

Drizzle with extra olive oil, if needed.

Musing No. 4
Start your day with a plan to eat a rainbow of colors.

HOMEMADE "MUSE" LI CEREAL

serves 2 - 4

There is something about the taste of muesli that makes me feel like some flower child at Woodstock. It's a feeling I quite like! This is a simple one that seems to work with me. You may, however, want to put your spin on it by using different seeds, nuts, or dried fruits.

1 ½ cups walnuts, finely chopped
2 cups rolled oats
½ cup pumpkin seeds
½ cup sunflower seeds
½ cup golden raisins or regular raisins
½ cup dried cranberry
1 ½ tablespoons turbinado sugar

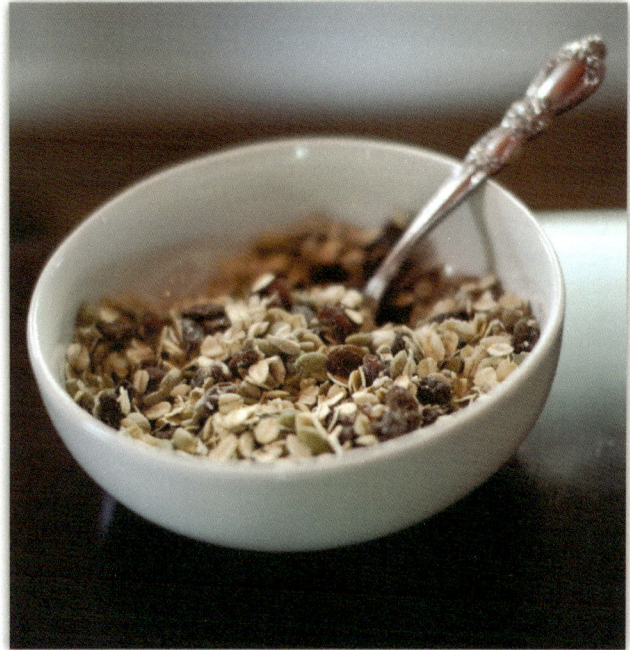

Preheat oven to 350 °F.

Spread chopped walnuts, oats, pumpkin seeds, and sunflower seeds on baking sheet and toast for about 25 minutes. After about 10 minutes, take out and shake mix so that it toasts evenly; place back into oven.

Once mix has toasted and cooled, add the raisins and cranberries. Sprinkle with turbinado.

Store in airtight container.

Musing No. 5

Set medjool dates out in the sunlight to warm then spread out the goodness onto toast for instant un-store bought jelly.

THE QUEEN'S QUINOA MUFFINS

makes 12 muffins

When you first think of muffins, they seem non-pretentious and rustic. By simply adding a bit of the "queen spice" cardamom to these, it evokes a layer of otherworldly richness which really is the charming thing about them!

1 cup white whole wheat or whole wheat pastry flour
⅔ cup raw cane sugar
1 tablespoon baking powder, aluminum free
1 teaspoon ground cardamom
½ teaspoon ground cinnamon
½ teaspoon ground ginger
1 cup coconut butter
⅔ cup almond milk
2 teaspoons pure vanilla extract
⅔ cup quinoa, cooked and cooled
½ cup cranberries
½ cup walnuts, chopped

Preheat the oven to 350°.

Generously coat muffin tin with coconut oil.

In a large bowl, combine flour, sugar, baking powder, cardamom, cinnamon, and ginger. In a separate bowl, mix coconut butter, milk, and vanilla.

Combine the wet and dry ingredients. Fold in the quinoa, cranberries, and walnuts being careful not to over mix. Divide the batter equally among the muffin cups.

For added sweetener, sprinkle turbinado over top of each muffin before baking. Bake for 20-25 min. or until a fork inserted into center comes out clean.

Musing No. 6

Create a ritual of honoring the morning light…with a quick set of sun-salutations outdoors before breakfast.

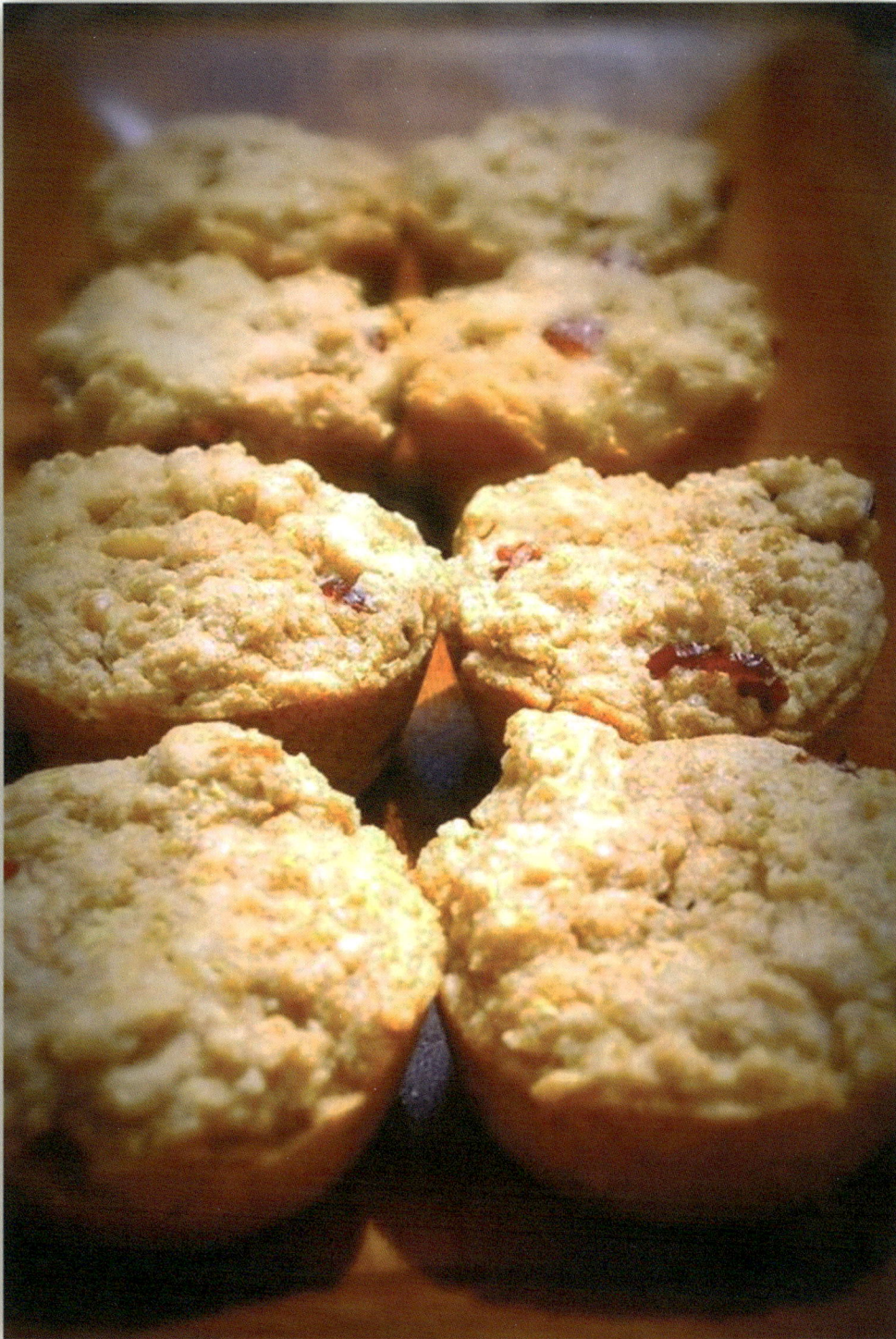

Musing No. 7

Try Yerba Maté instead of coffee to get you going in the a.m.

ROASTED ASPARAGUS WITH TOFU SCRAMBLE

serves 4 - 6

A tofu dish can seem mundane and ordinary at times, so think of the impact you want to create. Finding inspiration in seasonal vegetables and their colors, flavors, and textures can be an interesting way to approach your next tofu creation. I was drawn to the heat of the chili and its red color, the earthy taste of the asparagus, and the mustard hue of the turmeric. It's all about improvisation and intuitive inspirations. This could, of course, be crowned with just about any seasonal roasted vegetable that you have taken a liking to, so just use your muse-ment.

2 pounds fresh asparagus
extra virgin olive oil
1 ½ teaspoon sea salt
fresh ground pepper to taste

Preheat oven to 400 °F.

Snap off the tougher ends of the asparagus. Place on a baking sheet, drizzle with olive oil, sprinkle with sea salt and pepper, and then toss well. Spread in a single layer and roast for about 15 minutes until tender but still crisp.

While the asparagus is roasting, begin your tofu scramble.

TOFU SCRAMBLE

1 block firm organic tofu, pressed to get rid of excess water *(see note below)*
1 tablespoon extra virgin olive oil
2 - 4 tablespoons vegan butter
1 ½ teaspoons red pepper flakes
1 red bell pepper, diced
2 teaspoons shoyu
½ teaspoon turmeric
2 shallots, thinly sliced
1 clove garlic, minced
sea salt and fresh ground pepper to taste
one handful fresh cilantro, finely chopped (optional)

Drizzle olive oil in skillet pan over medium high heat. When the pan is warm, add the vegan butter followed by the pressed tofu.

With a spatula, chop and mash the tofu into scrambled egg-type pieces. Add the red pepper flakes, red bell pepper, shoyu, turmeric, shallots, and garlic. The tofu should begin to resemble the texture of scrambled eggs and also take on a yellow hue.

Cook over medium heat until the rest of the water has evaporated, tasting as you go. An additional sprinkle of turmeric to add in a deeper yellow is up to your discretion.

This should only take about 5 -10 minutes to prepare. Season with salt and pepper. Top it off with the fresh cilantro if desired.

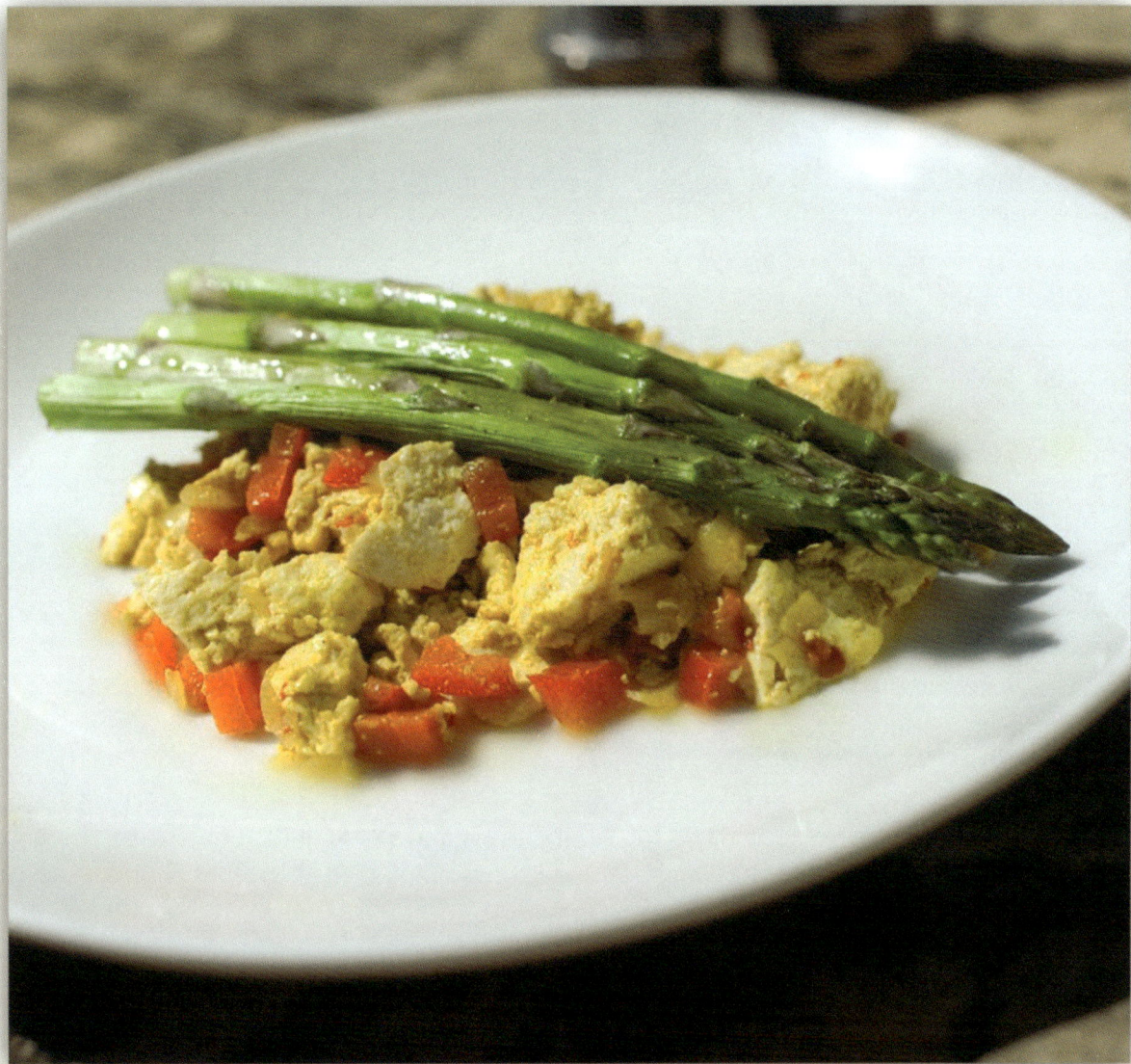

Musing No. 8

Parsley is also known as "the jewel of herbs." This jewel is not just for adorning your plates but is also a good source of folic acid and is one of the most important source for B vitamins.

TARTINE BREAKFAST SANDWICH
CROWNED WITH ROYAL PEPPER RELISH

serves 4

tartine (ta:'ti:n)
an open faced sandwich embellished with elaborate toppings.

I adore tartines (my newest obsession). Recently, I went through my stash of sandwich ideas and tweaked them a bit. Well, actually, I just turned them all into tartines! It is fun to eat sandwiches this way, and I feel less stuffed with the elimination of the extra bread. It's not so hard to take a classic, such as a breakfast sandwich, and update it a bit so it feels like a special occasion. These open-faced toasted gems are proper enough for royalty!

1 package firm organic tofu, drained well
1 tablespoon Bragg's Liquid Aminos
¼ teaspoon turmeric
sea salt and fresh ground pepper to taste
1 tablespoon extra virgin olive oil
4 whole wheat English muffins

Mix tofu, Bragg's Liquid Aminos, turmeric, sea salt, and pepper in a bowl using a fork to mash tofu into small pieces.

Preheat skillet over medium high heat. Drizzle skillet pan with olive oil. Add tofu mix, and cook until lightly browned on both sides. Turn heat to low and keep warm.

Prepare the Royal Pepper Relish listed below. Toast English muffins.

Using a spatula to lift tofu mix, place on top of open-faced toasted English muffins. With a large spoon, heap on the Royal Pepper Relish. Season with sea salt and fresh ground pepper to taste.

ROYAL PEPPER RELISH

½ red or yellow bell pepper, diced
2 garlic cloves, minced
½ red onion, diced
3 tablespoons fresh basil, chopped
4 tablespoons extra virgin olive oil
1 ½ tablespoons organic apple cider vinegar

In a small mixing bowl add in bell pepper, garlic, onion, basil, oil, and apple cider vinegar. Toss well and sprinkle with sea salt and ground pepper to taste.

Turmeric is also known as "The Golden Goddess." This golden spice has magnificent medicinal values. It is used as an antioxidant, antibiotic, and anti-inflammatory.

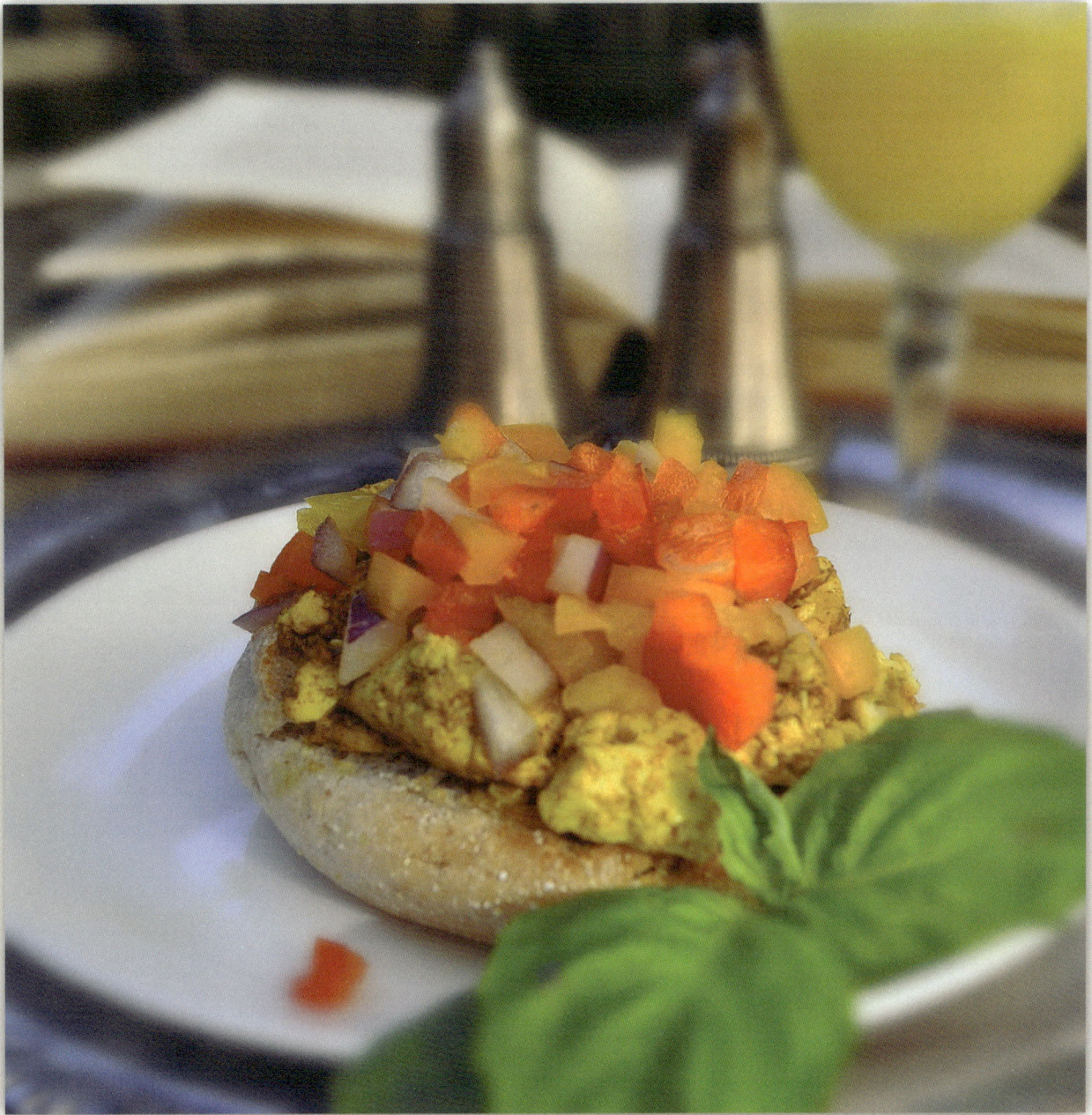

THE QUEEN'S QUINOA
serves 4

When a new season arrives, my imagination seems to kick into high gear, and the intrigue of quinoa is an open invitation for my mind to run wild. What seasonal fruit is beckoning you? Use this recipe as is or incorporate your favorite nuts and fresh fruits. This is truly my favorite breakfast. It's my nutrient-rich, whole grain goodness...my joie de vivre!

1 cup organic quinoa, pre-rinsed
1 cup coconut or almond milk
½ cup water
½ teaspoon sea salt
⅓ cup slivered almonds, toasted
½ teaspoon cardamom
1 banana, sliced
¼ cup golden raisins
¼ cup pure maple syrup

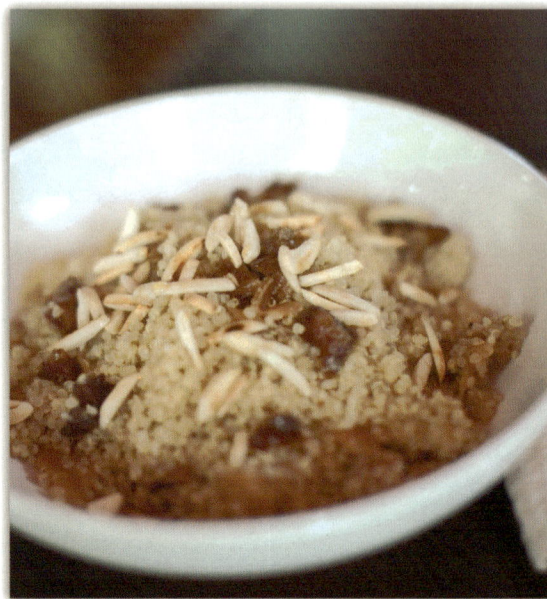

Soak quinoa for about 10-15 minutes. This will help the quinoa cook evenly and makes for a smoother taste as the soaking process helps to loosen the outer coating which can give a bitter taste.

Combine milk, water, quinoa, and salt in a medium saucepan. Bring to a boil. Reduce heat; cover and simmer for about 15 minutes or until most of the liquid is absorbed. Turn off heat; let quinoa stand covered for 5 minutes. Fluff quinoa gently with a fork.

Heat a dry skillet, and toast almonds over medium heat for about 2 - 3 minutes.
In separate bowl, combine cardamom, bananas, and golden raisins. Fold in the quinoa.
Sprinkle with toasted almonds, and drizzle with maple syrup.

Musing No. 10

Cardamom is known as "the queen of spices"...infuse more of this royal spice in your dishes.

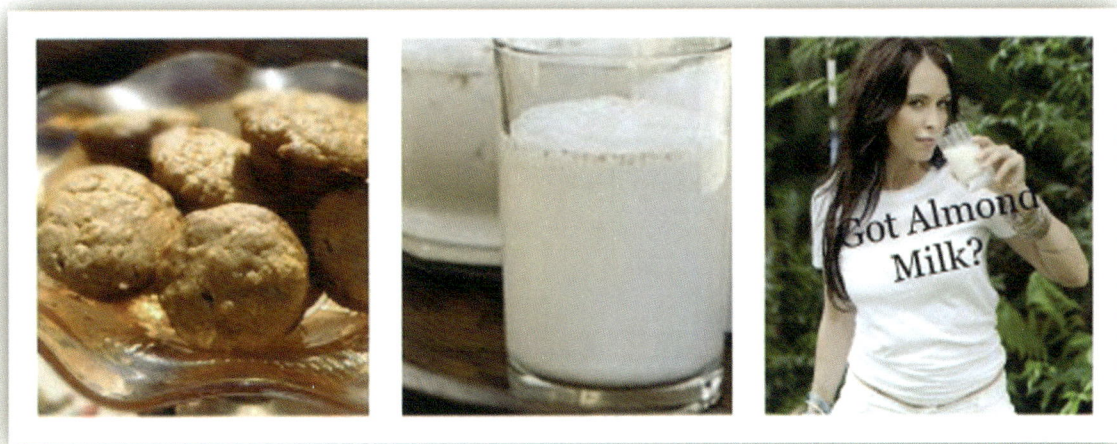

SWEET SPICED ALMOND MILK
makes ½ a gallon

As we are all busy, we reserve the right to cut corners here and there by purchasing store bought milks. Occasionally, I am right there with you in the line! However, I have made a point to set aside the time for making our own nut milks. This is really quite simple once you get into the habit. Whatever you create, enjoy the process and add your own spin on it.

1 cup raw almonds
7 ½ cups water
1 tablespoon brown rice syrup
1 teaspoon nutmeg

Put almonds in large bowl and cover almonds with water. Cover bowl with a cloth and place in a cool spot to soak for 24 hours. Drain off the water, rinse and put the almonds back into the bowl. Recover them with fresh water and soak for another 24 hours.

Drain off the water and put the plump almonds into a blender. Add 7 ½ cups water and blend. Add in brown rice syrup and nutmeg. Blend again.

Strain the milk through a sieve twice and pour the milk into a pitcher. Store in the refrigerator. Use within a week.

Musing No. 11
Add iron and fiber by using dried figs or apricots in your porridge.

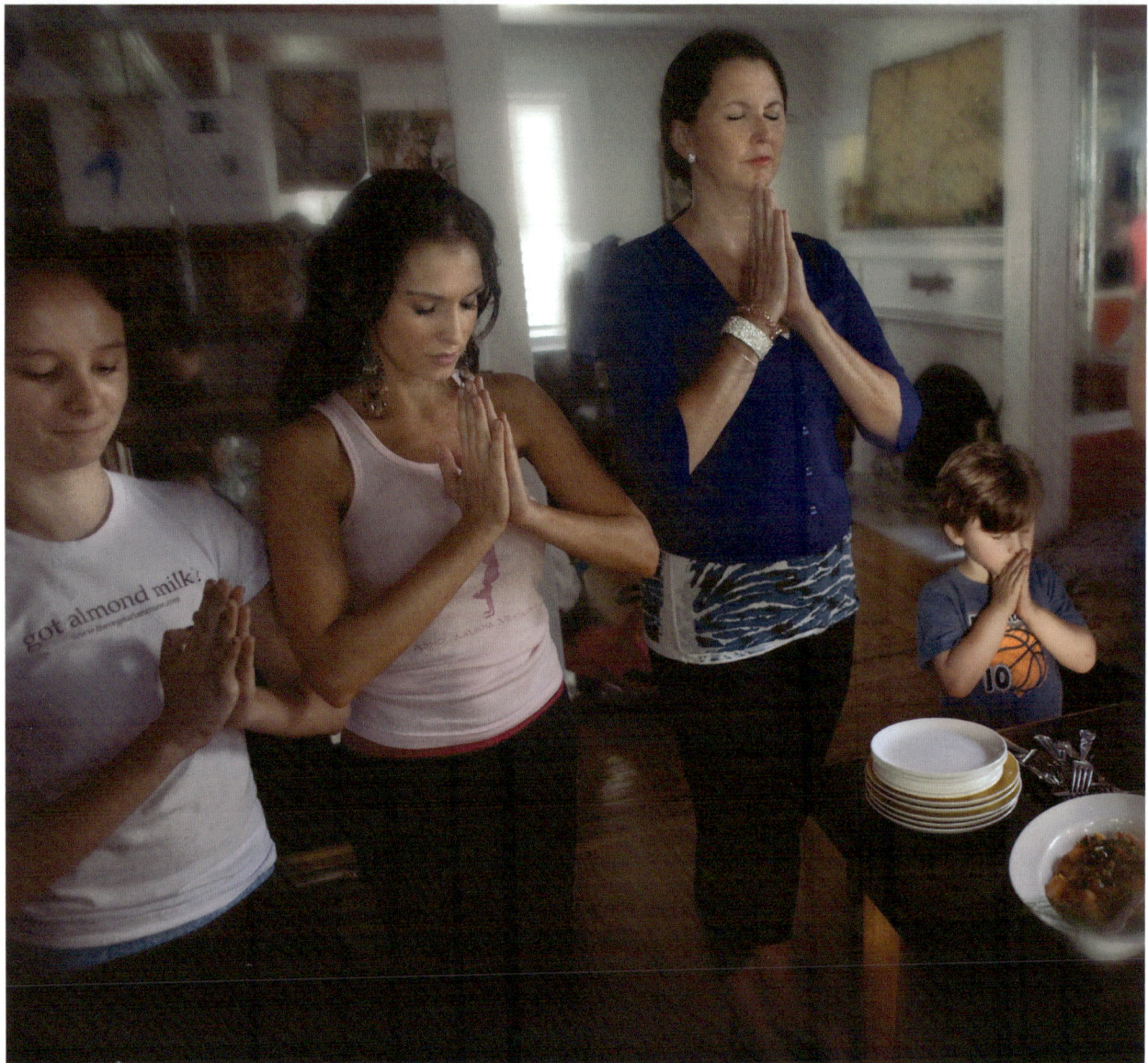

Musing No. 12

Mother Nature is a mysterious muse. Her glorious bounty provides a plethora of wonder to behold.

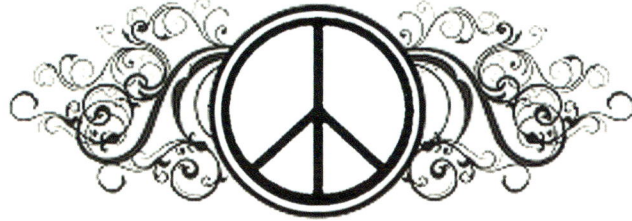

SANDWICHES & WRAPS

Really this section could be just as easily served as light dinners, I guess. I do love a good sandwich or wrap, so I am happy to have them anytime of day really! Peruse the soup and salad sections, mixing and matching - discovering your favorites.

TABOULEH TARTINE

serves 2

tartine (ta: 'ti:n)
an open faced sandwich embellished with elaborate toppings.

It's easy to add your own muse-ment to this gem of a sandwich. You could replace the pine nuts with almonds or pistachios and leave the mint out altogether. Although I find this to be perfect the way it is, you may want to work your creative magic with it.

½ cup fine bulgur
½ cup freshly squeezed lemon juice
¼ teaspoon agave nectar
1 cup pine nuts, toasted
1 ½ cups parsley, chopped finely
1 large tomato, diced
1 large cucumber, diced
5 scallions, chopped
½ cup fresh mint, finely chopped
4 - 6 tablespoons extra virgin olive oil
2 large sourdough or whole wheat bread slices, pre-toasted
sea salt and fresh ground pepper to taste

Pour bulgur in a bowl and cover with cold water. Soak for about 1 ½ hours until soft. Gently squeeze out excess water. Just spoon bulgur onto a clean kitchen towel, hold over sink, and squeeze.

Put bulgur in a medium saucepan, covering with fresh water and bring to a boil. Reduce heat and let stand for about 5 minutes.

Stir in lemon juice and agave nectar. Fluff with fork.

Add in the nuts, parsley, tomato, cucumber, scallions, mint, and oil.

Place in fridge for about two hours and allow to marinade.

Place a large spoonful of this goodness onto pre-toasted bread. Sprinkle sea salt and pepper to your liking.

Musing No. 13

Share lunch with Mother Nature. Eat outdoors more.

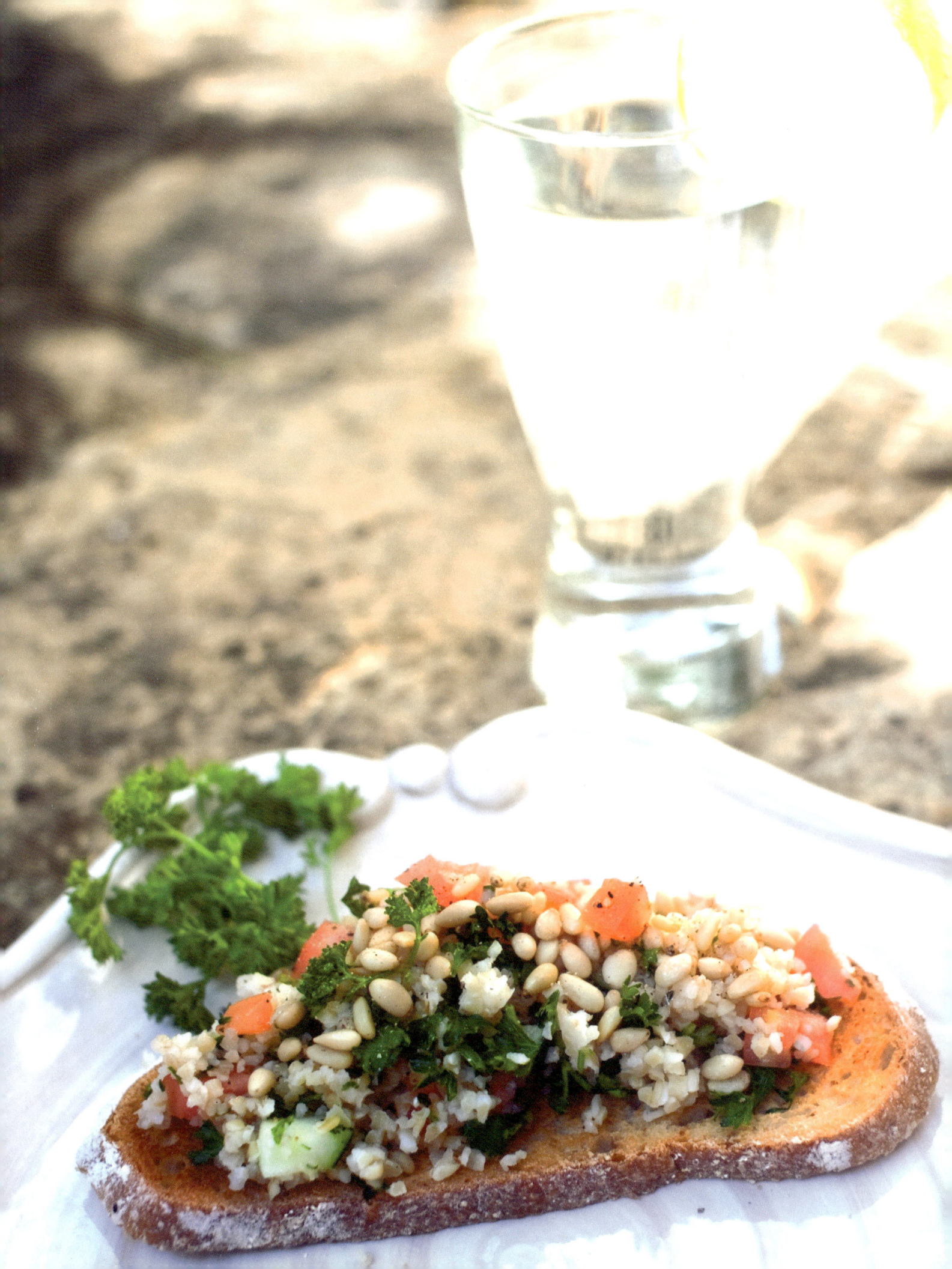

BOK CHOY SHITAKE WRAPS
serves 6

Enjoy the journey of life, the wonders of the many different cultures, and the plethora of ingredients available for food. Feed your imagination with a variety of recipes for your repertoire, and find time to learn about those ingredients that will add layers of flavors to your dishes.

3 tablespoons sesame oil
½ pound shitake mushrooms, julienne style
¾ pound baby bok choy, julienne style
3 medium carrots, julienne style
4 scallions, thinly sliced
1 tablespoon balsamic vinegar
2 teaspoons mirin
2 tablespoons shoyu
2 cloves garlic, minced
5 ounces pre-smoked tofu, sliced thin
sea salt and fresh ground pepper to taste
6 whole wheat tortillas, warmed and covered with a towel

Heat a sesame oil-coated skillet over high heat and sauté mushrooms for about 5 minutes or until softened.

Stir in bok choy, carrots, and scallions. Drizzle in balsamic vinegar, and cook for about 3 minutes. Add in mirin, shoyu, and garlic, and then sauté for about 1 more minute.

Add tofu; cook for 2 - 3 additional minutes or until heated, tossing carefully. Season with salt and pepper to taste. Spoon filling onto warmed tortillas. Fold into wraps.

Musing No. 14

For a spicy kick to your sandwiches or wraps...mix cayenne pepper, minced garlic & chopped cilantro to your vegan mayo.

AHIMSA-TUNA TEMPEH POCKETS
serves 4

Ahimsa - the first of the Yamas; non-violence, respecting all living creatures.
Yamas - ethical guidelines by which yogis/yoginis strive to live by.

Ever want to be like a Sea Shepherd and help protect the souls of the sea? Try this as a replacement for tuna salad. You are sure to feel a great ocean of consciousness begin. By making what may seem to be small adjustments in your lifestyle, you will, in fact, be a part of a greater cause.

3 tablespoons extra virgin olive oil
16 ounces tempeh, crumbled
2 tablespoons Bragg's Liquid Aminos
¼ cup celery, finely chopped
¼ cup scallions, finely chopped
¼ cup sunflower seeds
½ teaspoon fresh garlic, finely minced
1 teaspoon ground cumin
1 teaspoon dry dill weed
2 tablespoons flat-leafed Italian parsley, chopped
2 tablespoons lemon juice
1 cup vegan mayo
4 whole wheat pita pockets, sliced in half
8 cups fresh baby spinach
1 cucumber, thinly sliced
2 - 3 tablespoons vegan butter
sea salt and fresh ground pepper to taste

Drizzle olive oil onto skillet. Add tempeh crumbles, drizzle with Bragg's, stir well, and cook over medium-high heat for about 5 minutes until browned. Remove from heat and allow to cool.

In mixing bowl combine celery, scallions, sunflower seeds, garlic, cumin, dill weed, parsley, and lemon juice. Fold in vegan mayo and mix well.

Line each pita pocket with baby spinach, spoon in heaping amount of mayo mixture, then line with cucumber slices.

Reheat skillet over medium-high heat. Add vegan butter. When melted, carefully place a pre-stuffed pita onto pan and sear until crispy on each side.

Musing No. 15
Never, never, never run out of whole grains!

THE DAGWOOD TLT
serves 4

There is nothing lovelier or more calming than sitting in the shade with your family or friends and having a relaxing, no-fuss lunch. What will we have for lunch today? I say TLT's (Tempeh, Lettuce, and Tomato) and a nip of wine. My grandmother, Eva, was from the mountains of North Carolina where women lunched in hats and sun dresses. It makes me smile to think of her chatting with her friends while sipping her cool, refreshing glass of sweet sun-tea. How wonderful it must have been for her! In the summer, the mountain folk have long lunches, especially during the weekend. They unwind and take time to remember what's really important in life: dear friends, divine food, and blissful moments. What could be better? We can all live by this simple mantra and love life's little magical moments a bit more.

3 tablespoons olive oil
¼ cup shoyu
2 tablespoons balsamic vinegar
2 tablespoons pure maple syrup
8 ounces of tempeh, cut into 1/3- inch strips
⅓ cup vegan mayo
1 tablespoon lemon juice
1 tablespoon chopped parsley
½ teaspoon sea salt
¼ teaspoon ground black pepper
12 sourdough bread slices, toasted
2 - 3 cups mixed greens
2 cups alfalfa sprouts
2 tomatoes, sliced
2 avocados, peeled, seeded and sliced
1 medium onion, sliced

Whisk together oil, shoyu, vinegar, and syrup. Pour about half of this marinade into an 8x8 baking dish. Place tempeh in a single layer in baking dish. Pour marinade on top of the tempeh. Cover and marinade for about 30 minutes.

Preheat oven to 350 °F.

Pre-oil a baking sheet. Place the marinated tempeh onto baking sheet and bake for about 10-12 minutes. Flip tempeh over and bake for another 10-12 minutes. Remove and cool.

In small bowl, mix the vegan mayo, lemon juice, parsley, salt, and pepper.

Toast bread. Spread one bread slice evenly with the mayo mixture side up. Layer on some of the mixed greens, sprouts, tomato, avocado, onion slices. Top off with a layer of the marinated tempeh slices. Repeat again for second layer. Top with remaining bread slice. Repeat three more times to create all four sandwiches.

ASIAN INSPIRED TARTINE
serves 6

tartine (taːˈtiːn)
an open faced sandwich embellished with elaborate toppings.

My family and I have a thing for mouthwatering, sandwiches. We are forever creating combinations that make our lunches feel like works of art. We especially love the sort of sandwich that your fingers sink into, the kind that makes you break out your knife and fork! I had to share this recipe with you because I want you to experience a vegan sandwich that is hearty, rich in nutrients, and ready for your own mused touches. Just keep in mind that you will need to have a huge cloth napkin handy for all the divine drippings! I love this with a hot tea and sliced ginger. It seems to tame my Asian inspired daydreams.

¼ cup shoyu
2 tablespoons raw cane sugar
2 tablespoons fresh ginger, minced
2 cloves garlic, minced
3 - 4 tablespoons of water
1 10-ounce package firm tofu, drained well and cut into 12 slices
2 cups bean sprouts
1 cucumber, thinly sliced
½ red onion, thinly sliced
½ cup sesame seeds, toasted
3 tablespoons sesame oil
6 slices sourdough or whole wheat bread, ½ - inch thick, toasted

Combine shoyu, sugar, ginger, and garlic in bowl. Mix in water. Add tofu slices, and coat each slice well. Allow this to set for about 20 minutes, so the tofu can fully envelope the flavors. Remove tofu and reserve marinade mixture.

Combine sprouts, cucumber, onion, and sesame seeds in a separate bowl, and pour reserved marinade mix overtop. Coat well.

Drizzle skillet with sesame oil and heat over medium-high temperature. Sauté tofu, until both sides are slightly browned.

Toast bread slices. Top each slice with two slices of tofu.

Pile coated veggies onto each open-faced sandwich.

Musing No. 16

Snack on sea veggies, toasted seeds, and leftover brown rice.

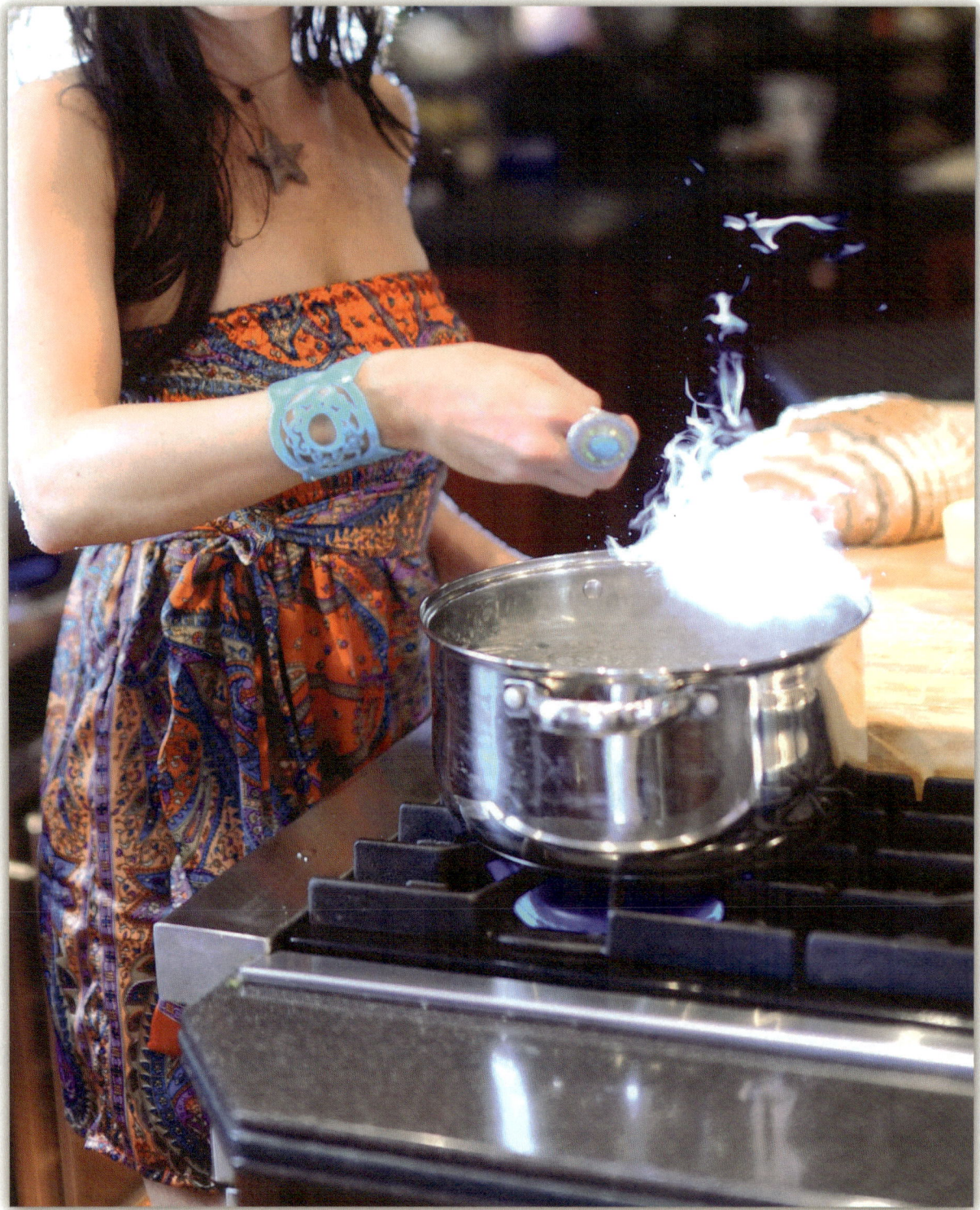

Musing No. 17

Feel cozy and warm on a crisp cold eve with the moonlight and a bowl of warm bliss.

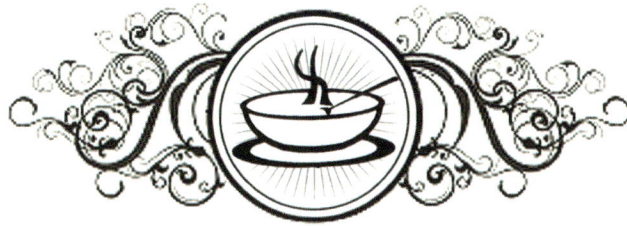

SOUPS

Greet your meal with the warmest welcome. Mix your kitchen secrets with compassionate culinary concoctions. That is a surefire way to bring harmony to your mind, warm nourishment to your body, and instant soothing to your soul.

SACRED SOUP
serves 6

Inspired by the Sacral Chakra...which is said to have an orange hue. The Sacral Chakra represents vitality and promotes emotional balance, health, and pleasure. The earthiness of the carrot is the star attraction in this inspired, soul-soothing, spirit-lifting soup. While the ginger and garlic evokes a pungent aromatic layer. The subtle layers of sweet potato, onion, and spices strike an exotic note. The sweetness of coconut milk and brown rice syrup pulls this courtship of flavors together. The sacral chakra, which has an orange hue, represents vitality and promotes emotional balance, health, and pleasure.

1 tablespoon extra virgin olive oil
1 onion, chopped
3 cloves garlic, chopped
2 tablespoons chopped fresh ginger
1 ½ teaspoon ground cumin
1 ½ teaspoon paprika
a pinch cayenne
1 ½ pound carrots, chopped
1 large sweet potato, peeled chopped
6 cups veggie stock
1 cup coconut milk
1 tablespoon brown rice syrup
1 tablespoon fresh squeezed lime juice
sea salt and fresh ground pepper to taste
cilantro, finely chopped

Heat olive oil in a large saucepan over medium heat. Add onion, garlic, and ginger. Cook gently until fragrant - about 5 minutes. Stir in cumin, paprika, and cayenne. Cook for about a minute until fragrant. Add carrots, sweet potato, veggie stock, coconut milk, brown rice syrup, and lime juice.

Cook 30 - 40 minutes until vegetables are very tender. Puree soup and reheat. Season with salt and pepper to taste.

Garnish with chopped cilantro and grated carrots and serve.

Musing No. 18

There are no two soups completely alike. They are, by nature, quaint in their own right and warm the soul like no other...

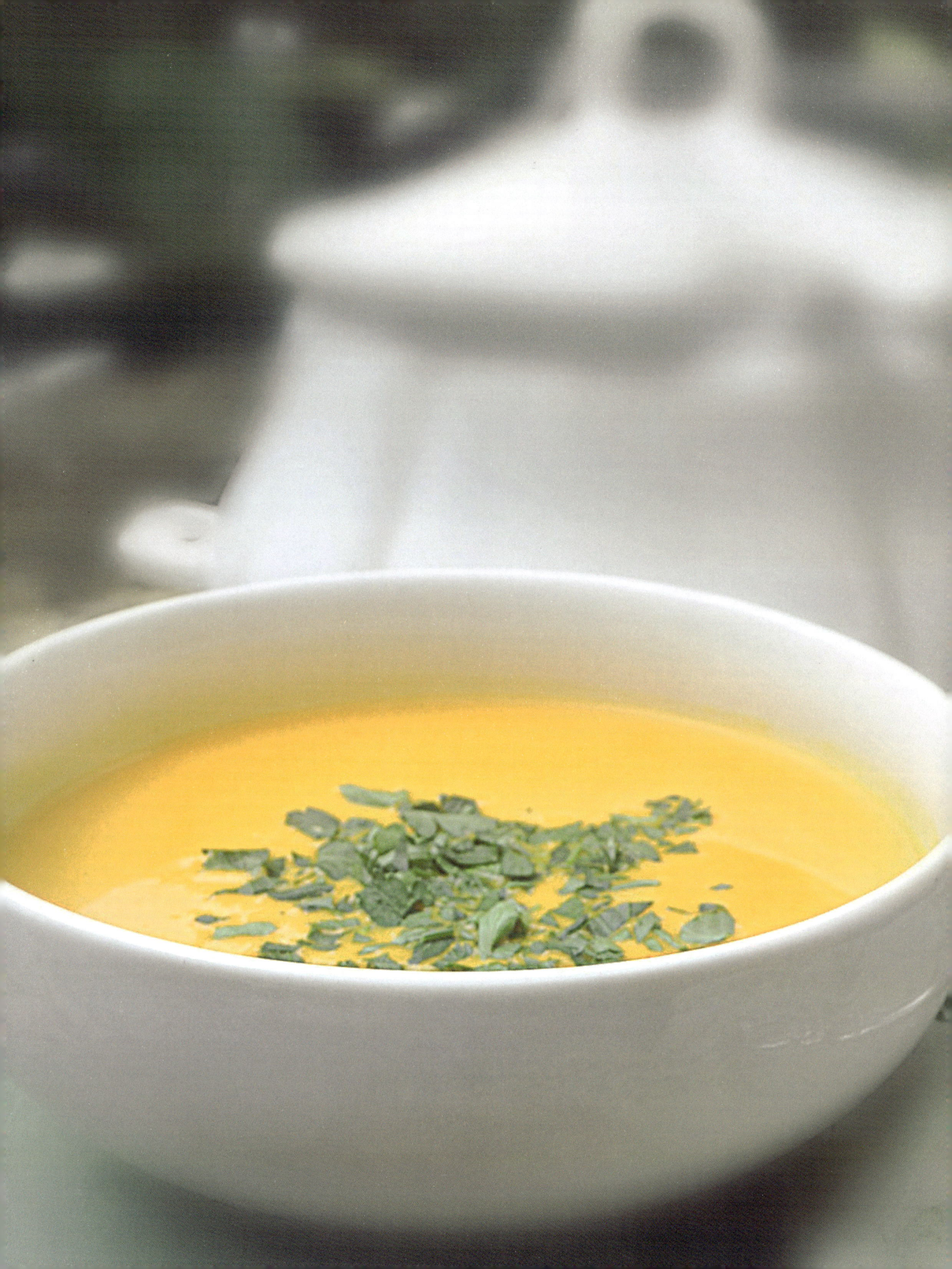

ROASTED RED PEPPER AND AVOCADO GAZPACHO
serves 4

Avocados have a nickname that my kids love... alligator pears! There's so much goodness to love about a good gazpacho. Gazpachos come in many variations and dimensions, are highly personal, and everyone loves them.

2 ½ cups plum tomatoes, chopped
1 cucumber, chopped
2 red bell peppers, roasted and chopped
2 scallions, chopped
¼ cup whole cilantro
2 tablespoons whole parsley
1 tablespoon balsamic vinegar
1 tablespoon fresh squeezed lemon juice
2 tablespoons extra virgin olive oil
1 avocado, peeled and pitted, divided
1 teaspoon fresh ground pepper
1 teaspoon sea salt

In a blender, add tomatoes, cucumber, red peppers, scallions, cilantro, parsley, vinegar, lemon juice, olive oil, one half of the avocado, pepper, and salt. Blend until well-combined but still has a slightly chunky consistency

Cover, and chill in refrigerator for 2 hours to allow flavors to envelope.

Chop remaining avocado to garnish top of gazpacho for each serving.

Musing No. 19
*Serve cold gazpachos in hollowed avocado shells...
great for a unique soup bowl.*

Musing No. 20
*Want a creamier soup base? Try blending one cup of soup stock with
one quarter cup of tofu. Stir well and add back into soup pot. Viola!*

THE SHAMAN'S SOUP

serves 6

Give your soup a plethora of healing ingredients that have depth and flavor. The miso is a known regulator of women's estrogen and is rich with antioxidants. The seaweed, nori, is rich in iodine, iron, and protein and is linked to lowering the risk of breast cancer. The shiitake mushroom is used in traditional Oriental medicine to prevent high blood pressure and heart disease. These ingredients combined will offer you their doses of healing magic for whatever is ailing you.

8 cups veggie stock
4 cloves garlic, minced
4 ounces shiitake mushrooms,
   stems discarded, caps thinly sliced
2 small carrots, thinly sliced
⅓ cup cilantro, finely chopped
⅓ cup watercress
3 tablespoons shoyu
2 tablespoons sesame oil
pinch of red pepper flakes
2 - 4 tablespoons miso paste to taste
1 ½ tablespoons shredded nori
4 scallions, thinly sliced
sea salt and fresh ground pepper to taste

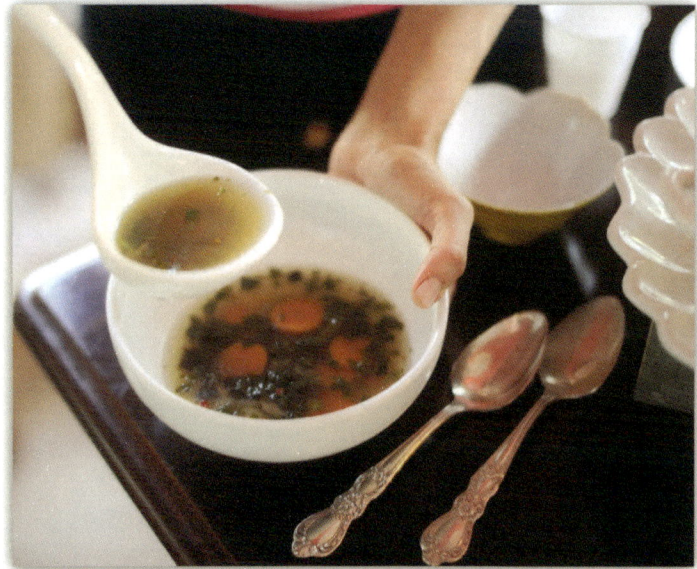

In a stock pot, mix veggie stock, garlic, mushrooms, carrots, cilantro, watercress, shoyu, sesame oil, and red pepper flakes. Bring to a boil, the turn down heat and simmer 15 - 20 minutes.

In a small bowl, scoop out a bit of the of the soup stock from the pot, and dissolve the miso paste in it using a wooden spoon. Gradually add the miso mixture back into the soup. Stir the soup gently. Do not boil the miso because it seems to change the flavor and will also remove some of the healthy properties.

Add the nori seaweed. Allow to simmer at least 5 - 6 minutes. The longer you simmer the sea veggie, the less of a salty, fishy flavor it will have. Turn off the stove and add the chopped scallions. Salt and pepper to taste. Serve

Musing No. 21

Personalize your soups. Sauté one half cup aromatics (fennel, onions, and celery) and 2 cloves garlic in a bit of olive oil until softened. Crown your soups with this. It will take an austere soup and give it instant flair!

BOHO SOUP AND DUMPLINGS
serves 6-8

This soup is somewhat informal, hence the name Boho Soup. Boho is the nick to the name bohemian. Although the bohemian culture is well known for living an unconventional life, the creative talents of art, music, and writing seems to take the informal way of their lifestyle to a level of allure. The allure to this simple, rustic, yet spellbinding soup is its mild bean base. It holds its spectacular texture once you load it up with all the lovely layers of herbs, veggies, dumplings and simple goodness!

BOHO SOUP

1 ½ cups drained white beans (presoaked overnight)
1 bay leaf
6 tablespoons olive oil
4 shallots, finely chopped
1 large leek, finely chopped
1 carrot, thinly chopped
6 cups water
6 cups veggie stock
1 tablespoon tahini
1 splash white wine
3 cloves garlic, minced
2 slices of ginger root, minced
2 medium tomatoes, diced
4 tablespoons rosemary, finely chopped
sea salt and fresh ground pepper to taste
2 tablespoons vegan butter
2 tablespoons extra virgin olive oil

1 handful fresh parsley, chopped

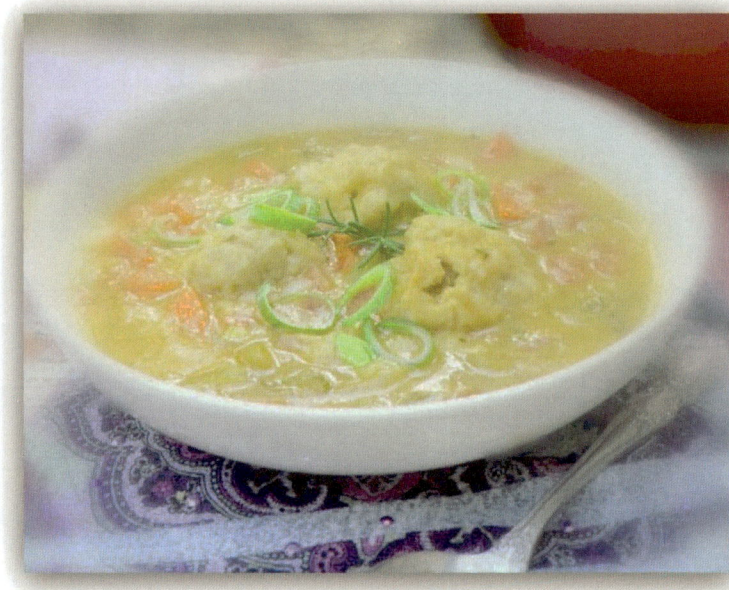

Place beans in a large saucepan of water. Bring to a boil. Cook for about 25 minutes. Drain. Return beans to pot, and cover with cool water. Bring to a second boil. Add bay leaf, and cook until beans are tender (1 ½ to 2 hours). Drain beans again. Remove bay leaf.

In a skillet, heat oil, and stir in the shallots; cook until soft. Add the leek and carrot; cook for

about 5 minutes. Pour in the water and veggie stock. Add tahini, wine, garlic, and ginger. Stir well. Add in tomatoes and rosemary. Sprinkle sea salt and pepper to taste. Add the vegan butter and stir. Reduce to low heat.

Make Dumplings.

Bring to a low boil, and add dollops of the dumplings. Drop the dough in spoonfuls into the broth. Cover the pot and reduce to simmer. Cook for 10 - 15 minutes, just until dumplings are cooked. Do not overcook.

Drizzle with a little olive oil, and add fresh parsley. Season to taste.

DUMPLINGS

¾ cup hemp milk
1 teaspoon brown rice vinegar
2 cups white whole wheat flour
1 tablespoon baking powder, aluminum free
½ teaspoon sea salt
¼ cup vegan butter

Mix the milk and vinegar, and set aside for a few minutes.

In a bowl, combine the flour, baking powder, and salt. Cut in the vegan butter until crumbly. Add the milk and vinegar mixture and stir until a dough like consistency is formed.

Musing No. 22

Don't be too formal when serving soup. For an eclectic bohemian ambiance… mix and match your soup bowls, napkins, and, of course, conversation.

Musing No. 23

Garlic, a well known companion of soup, has been used since ancient times and is a symbol of vitality. Garlic, garlic, garlic. Don't forget the garlic!

DEEPLY ROOTED SOUP

serves 6

I'm drawn to vegetables grown underground. I find them otherworldly and full of mystery. They drink in the nutrients from the dark underground, transform perfectly into magic roots of nutrition, and have the most beautiful earthy colors. I heard once they are the soul of plants. This soup is something I crave now and then.

¼ cup vegan butter
2 large sweet potatoes, chopped and cubed
1 parsnip, chopped and cubed
1 apple, chopped and cubed
3 carrots, thinly chopped
3 celery sticks, thinly chopped
1 leek, thinly chopped
4 garlic cloves, minced
½ cup red lentils, pre-soaked
½ teaspoon fresh ginger, minced
1 teaspoon sea salt
½ teaspoon ground black pepper
A pinch of cumin
A pinch of paprika
4 cups veggie broth
4 cups water
2 bay leaves
fresh thyme sprigs (optional)

Melt vegan butter in a large soup pot over medium-high heat. Place sweet potatoes, parsnip, apple, carrots, celery, leek, and garlic in the pot. Stir and cook for about 10 minutes.

Pour in the lentils, ginger, salt, pepper, cumin, paprika, and veggie broth and water. Add bay leaves. Bring soup to a boil over high heat. Reduce heat, cover, and simmer for about 30- 35 minutes or until the lentils are soft. Remove bay leaves. Season with salt and pepper to taste, if desired. Garnish with fresh thyme sprigs, season with salt and pepper as desired.

Musing No. 24

Want a clever way to impress your guests? Serve an unforgettable savory soup before dinner that powers the prana within.

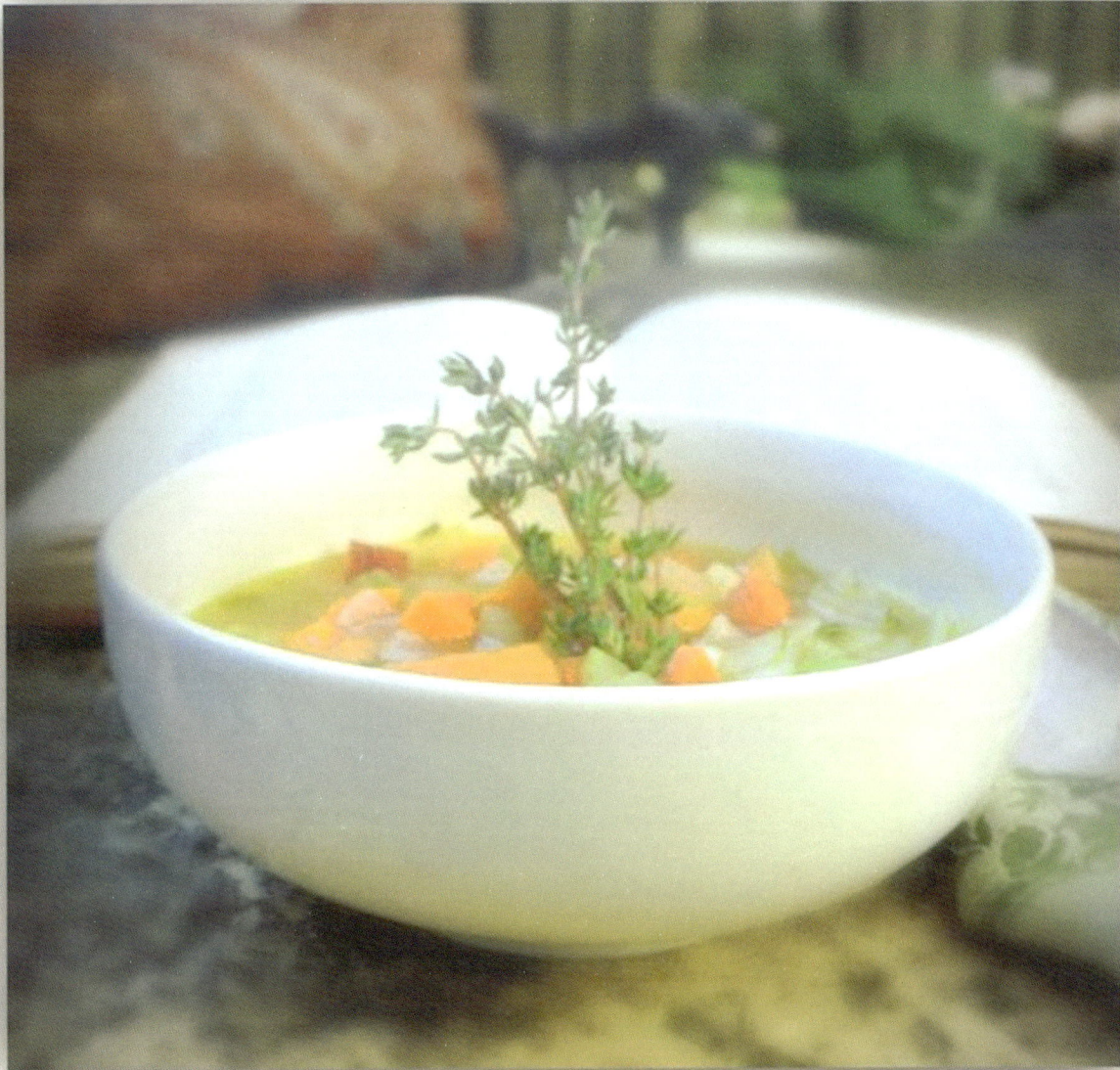

Musing No. 25

For soups & stews: always, always, always add a handful or two of herbs.

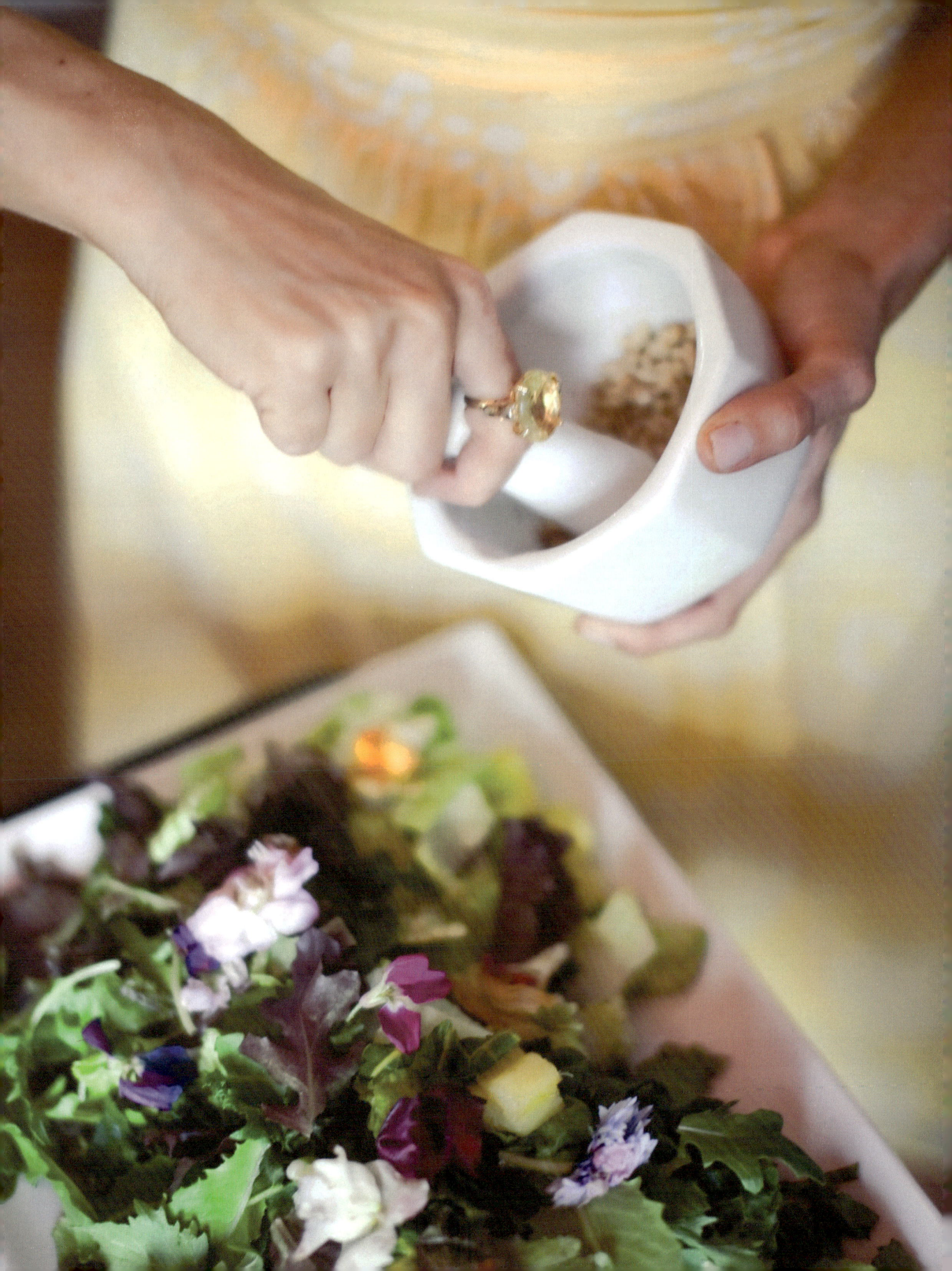

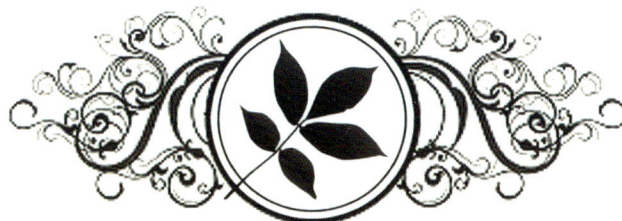

SALADS

A WELL-DRESSED SALAD IS A ONE-DISH WONDER AND ALWAYS SEEMS ADORN JUST ABOUT ANY MEAL. SO, IT IS A GOOD IDEA TO HAVE SOME YUMMY VINAIGRETTES AND DRESSINGS IN YOUR STASH. I HAVE OFFERED SOME QUICKIES TO WHIP UP WHEN YOU ARE LOOKING TO ADD THAT EXTRA LAYER OF FLAVOR. USE VINAIGRETTES AND CREAMY DRESSINGS TO MIX NOT ONLY IN YOUR SALADS BUT IN LEFTOVER RICE AND PASTA DISHES FOR AN ADDED ELEMENT THAT IS SURE TO EVOKE A MOST SERENDIPITOUS DISH.

THE RED SLAW

serves 6 - 8

Coleslaw is an American tradition, or at least it is in my family. Give yours a little twist with toasted sesame seeds, cilantro, and rice vinegar. For those in search of the perfect coleslaw, I highly recommend this one. I find that it is even better the next day. I also use this recipe as a garnish for our Sunday Portobello Burgers.

2 red chilies, finely chopped
2 cloves garlic, minced
1 red onion, shredded
2 pounds red cabbage, shredded
5 small radishes, sliced finely
1 bunch fresh cilantro, finely chopped
6 tablespoons sesame oil
6 tablespoons rice vinegar
3 tablespoons lime juice
2 tablespoons turbinado sugar
¼ cup vegan mayonnaise
sea salt and fresh ground pepper to taste
1 cup sunflower seeds, pre-toasted

When you finely chop the chilies, be careful to wash hands immediately.

In a large bowl, add chilies, garlic, red onion, red cabbage, radishes, and cilantro.

In a separate bowl, whisk together sesame oil, rice vinegar, lime juice, and sugar. Pour over top of slaw and mix well. Let marinate for about an hour.

Fold in vegan mayonnaise. Season with sea salt and pepper to taste. Add toasted sunflower seeds to top.

Musing No. 26

The large, solitary blossom of the sunflower is composed of a ray of yellow florets. These flowers are notable for turning their faces to the sun. This behavior is known as heliotropism. Just as the sunflower basks in the vitamin D of our sun, so should we. Find a moment to close your eyes, turn your face towards the sun, and feel its warm kiss.

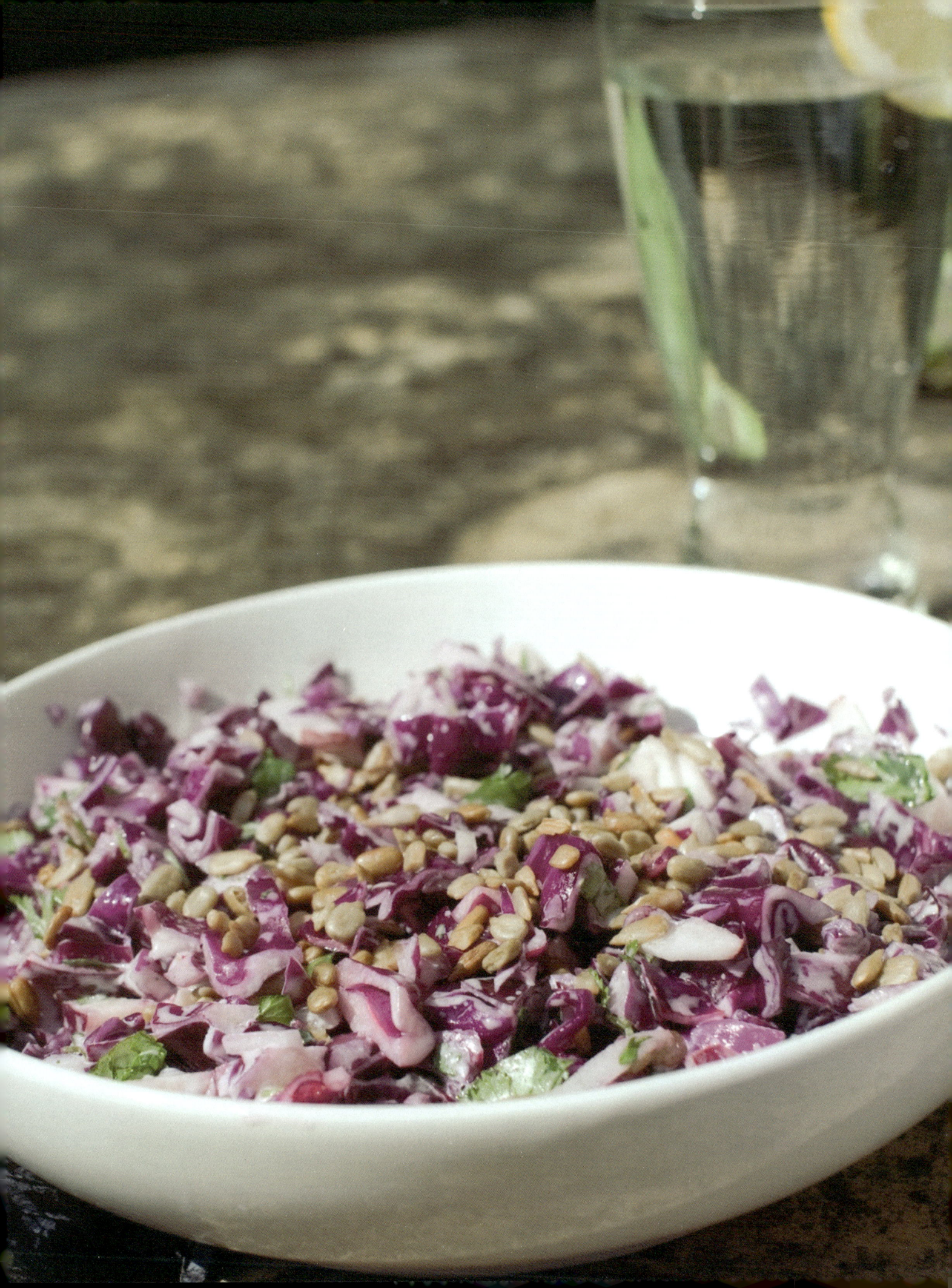

KALE AND ROASTED GARLIC SALAD

serves 4 - 6

Freshly picked veggies from your garden or from your local Farmers' Market are the best. When you are in a hurry, there's nothing better than reaching for what's outside your door or for what is local. There is no need to worry about the amount of garlic in this salad. When garlic is roasted, it becomes more subtle and sweet; it will loose its pungent taste. This is one of those stand-alone kinds of salad. No need for fancy dressings here! Just the simplicity of it is a wonder to behold!

1 pound kale, chopped
juice of ½ lemon
¼ cup extra virgin olive oil
½ cup sesame seeds, toasted
sea salt and fresh ground pepper to taste
12 garlic cloves, unpeeled

In a skillet over medium heat, add kale and flash cook it.

Preheat oven to 375 °F.

In a large salad bowl, add the kale and lemon juice. Massage well. Drizzle with olive oil. Toss well. Add toasted sesame seeds, sea salt, and pepper to taste.

In a roasting dish, place garlic and toss in olive oil. Bake for about 15 minutes. You will want the garlic to be slightly charred. While the garlic is still warm, add to the salad and toss.

Musing No. 27

In yoga and meditation, our focus becomes set on our third eye and heightened enlightenment. In our daily diet, our focus should become set on the health of our temple (body). Kale has numerous benefits of astounding proportions. The one I find interesting is its ability to protect our eyes by reducing the risk of cataracts. So whether your focus is set on your inner eye or on your outer eyes, the magic of kale is sure to lend its power.

WHITE BEAN AND ARTICHOKE SALAD
WITH CREAMY GARLIC DRESSING
serves 4 - 6

It's amazing how the white bean can go from austere to sensational with a mix of herbs and fresh greens. With the white bean or the cannelloni bean's mild flavor, it seems to be the perfect choice for most salad and soup creations.

3 cups white kidney beans, presoaked
½ cup diced red onion
1 tablespoon fresh minced rosemary
6 sun dried tomatoes, sliced
2 cans artichoke hearts, drained, rinsed, and quartered
1 ½ cups coarsely chopped fresh parsley
1 pound spring mix greens
¼ cup Creamy Garlic Dressing
sea salt and fresh ground pepper to taste
fresh parsley (optional)

TO SOAK:

Rinse beans. Place beans in pot and fill with water to cover by at least 4 inches. Soak white beans overnight. When ready to cook, drain beans and return to soup pot. Add enough water to cover beans by about 2 inches. Slowly bring to a boil. Reduce heat and simmer. Cook for about 1 ½ hours or until beans are tender but not mushy. Remove from heat, drain and cool.

In a separate bowl combine red onion, fresh minced rosemary, dried tomatoes, artichoke hearts, and chopped parsley.

In a large serving platter, place the spring mix.

Pour on creamy garlic dressing and mix well. Spoon bean mixture on top of greens. Sprinkle with salt, pepper, and fresh parsley (optional).

CREAMY GARLIC DRESSING

5 garlic cloves
3 ½ tablespoons brown rice vinegar
½ cup pine nuts
1 teaspoon thyme
1 teaspoon oregano
1 teaspoon sea salt
1 cup sourdough bread crumbs
½ cup water
5 - 6 tablespoons extra virgin olive oil

In a blender combine garlic, vinegar, nuts, thyme, oregano, salt, breadcrumbs, water, and oil. Blend until smooth.

POM-POM SALAD & AGAVE ORANGE VINAIGRETTE

serves 4

The pomegranate has long been a known muse for many poets, writers, and artists. Ancient myths say this fruit was favored by the gods. Its red colored seeds have a ruby, shiny, gem like appearance which some refer to as "winter jewels." But even these royal gems need a bit of gypsy love, hence paring it with the earthy, well traveled fennel bulb. Fennel is said to be indigenous to the shores of the Mediterranean. Fennel lends itself to many culinary creations as it is a highly aromatic plant. This sweet yet earthy salad offers much goodness to bring to the "altar" (table).

4 big handfuls of arugula
1 red onion, thinly sliced
½ teaspoon lemon peel, freshly grated
1 large fresh fennel bulb, trimmed, halved, thinly sliced
1 Fuji apple, diced
seeds of 4 pomegranates
Agave Orange Vinaigrette

Heap the arugula in a large salad bowl. Sprinkle on the sliced onion, grated lemon, fennel, and apple.

Just before serving, drizzle desired amount of the Agave Orange Vinaigrette and toss well. Scatter the "pom-pom" seeds on top.

AGAVE ORANGE VINAIGRETTE

½ cup organic orange juice
2 tablespoons brown rice syrup
½ tablespoon ginger
Pinch of sea salt
Fresh ground black pepper to taste
1 cup extra virgin olive oil

Mix orange juice and agave in a medium sized bowl and stir until agave dissolves into the orange juice. Add sea salt and pepper. Slowly stream in the olive oil as you whisk, until all is combined.

Heap the greens in a large salad bowl. Sprinkle on the minced onion. Then scatter the pomegranate seeds on top. Just before serving drizzle vinaigrette and toss well.

Musing No. 28
Remember, it's the little details that create the magic.

CANTALOUPE PEPPER SALAD

serves 6 - 8

When you learn to experiment with some rather unpredictable pairings, you'll find that voila moment. The idea is that a combination of varied elements enhances the dish. This combo seems to make a statement and creates an exotic paring on its own.

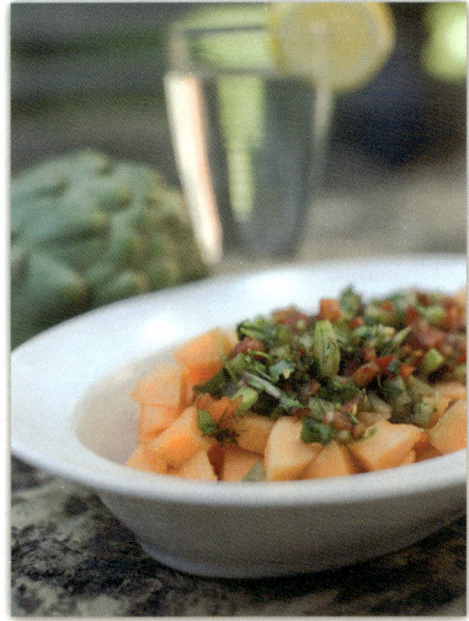

6 cloves of garlic, peeled
2 sticks celery, roughly chopped
1 red pepper, roughly chopped
½ cups fresh dill
1 ½ cups fresh cilantro, chopped
4 tablespoons organic red wine vinegar
¼ teaspoon sea salt
½ tablespoons red pepper flakes
2 green or cantaloupe melons, cubed

Put the peeled garlic, celery, and red pepper in a food processor, and pulse until almost minced. Or, if you are chopping by hand, just chop as finely as possible. Add the dill and cilantro into processor and pulse again until blended.

Place this mix into bowl, and add in the vinegar, salt, and red pepper flakes. Mix well. Place into a recycled jar or a mason jar, and let stand overnight.

Cut melons in half and cube. Place onto a large platter with the hot pepper salad in the middle. Garnish with fresh dill.

Musing No. 29

Vibrant colors, intricately woven flavors, and other dazzling details make your meals most excellent.

UTOPIAN LENTIL SALAD
serves 4

Take pleasure in the world. Enjoy the lovely buffet of wonder – life's feast -- in its beautifully divine simplicity. This goes for food as well. I would much rather create and enjoy a simple lunch that leaves me entirely satisfied rather than a plate piled high with junk. This is a simple salad that I have left open to your whim as far as the amounts of oil and vinegar go. I tend to add more or less depending on what I am in the mood for. The companionship of these simple elements joined together unites quite a marriage!

4 cups red lentils
juice of ½ lemon
1 pound kale chopped
1 red bell pepper
olive oil, as needed
ume plum vinegar to taste
sea salt, to taste
fresh ground pepper, to taste

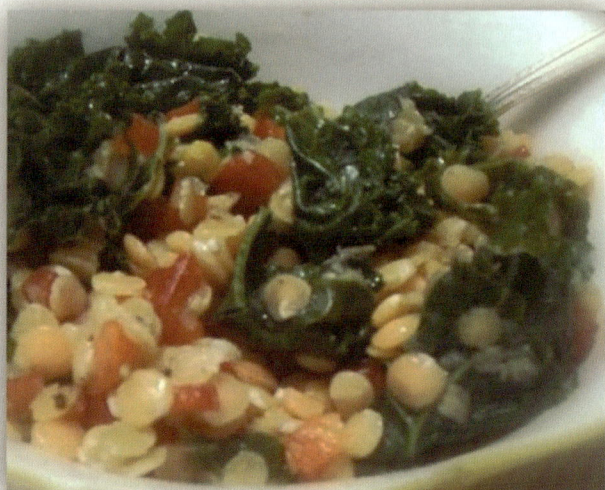

Soak lentils for about 3 hours. In a sauce pan, bring lentils to a boil or cook in pressure cooker until done.

While lentils are cooking, toss lemon juice and kale together. Massage well.

Preheat oven to 400 °F.

Slice red bell pepper and coat in olive oil. Place on a baking sheet and roast for about 30 minutes. Pull from oven, let cool, and then chop.

Put lentils into a salad bowl, drizzle some extra virgin olive oil over it, and mix. Drizzle in some ume plum vinegar, and mix. Add in kale, peppers, salt, and pepper to desired taste.

Musing No. 30

Garnishing can be another way to add layers of raw veggies, seeds, and nuts to the mix. Simple, crispy, crunchy, colorful, local, and seasonal tokens entice the eyes and nourish the body.

BULGUR SALAD EXTRAORDINAIRE
WITH THE GYPSY'S DRESSING
serves 2 - 4

I do love a quick, hearty salad. Okay, well I dig any salad, but the minute you add a creamy dressing to it, I am a certified spoon-licker extraordinaire. This salad is a quickie but is very tasty. You had better make more than you need, because you will want it on toast for a light snack or, better yet, an open-faced sandwich.

1 cup bulgur wheat
½ cup sliced mushrooms
2 tablespoons extra virgin olive oil
2 cups vegetable stock
2 green onions, chopped
2 cup finely shredded red cabbage
¼ cup of The Gypsy's Dressing (page 64)

Sauté bulgur wheat and mushrooms in olive oil until golden.

Add vegetable stock, cover, and bring to boil. Reduce heat and simmer 20 minutes. Allow to cool.

Toss cooled bulgur mixture with green onions, red cabbage, and The Gypsy's Dressing.

Musing No. 31

The gypsy's dressing offers the spirit lifting, energy enhancing herb, mint. For a quick energy boosting tea, check out the Shaman's Mint Tea on page 128.

AROMATIC HERBAL TOSS SALAD
serves 4

Usually I let the salad inspire the dressings that I drizzle on top of a mix of greens, but this is one of those that just seemed to form on its own! Using my mortar and pestle is just one of those things I enjoy about preparing foods! It makes me feel like an alchemist in my kitchen. Sometimes, just by dabbling with different herbs and such, you can come up with the most divine repast. My kids love to use the mortar and pestle as well, which seems to inspire them to create new tastes, thus enticing them to eat their creations.

6 cups mixed leaves: ruby chard, arugula, romaine, dandelion greens
½ cup basil, chopped
½ cup chives, chopped
½ cup parsley, chopped
¼ cup mint, chopped
edible flowers (optional)
⅓ cup extra virgin olive oil
4 tablespoons pine nuts
2 ½ teaspoons apple cider vinegar
sea salt and fresh ground pepper to taste

Put your assorted salad leaves and herbs in a large salad bowl and set aside.

In a skillet, heat olive oil and sauté pine nuts for about 5 minutes, until evenly golden. Let cool.

Using a mortar and pestle, smash and then grind pine nuts until they have a mushy consistency.

In a small bowl, add the ground pine nuts. Slowly whisk in olive oil and blend well. Add vinegar, salt, and pepper to taste and mix well. Pour over salad and with hands, toss well.

Musing No. 32

Try exploring this simple recipe with your favorite seeds, nuts and dried fruits. Be fearless in your own kitchen, try new things; explore new ways of integrating doses of creativity.

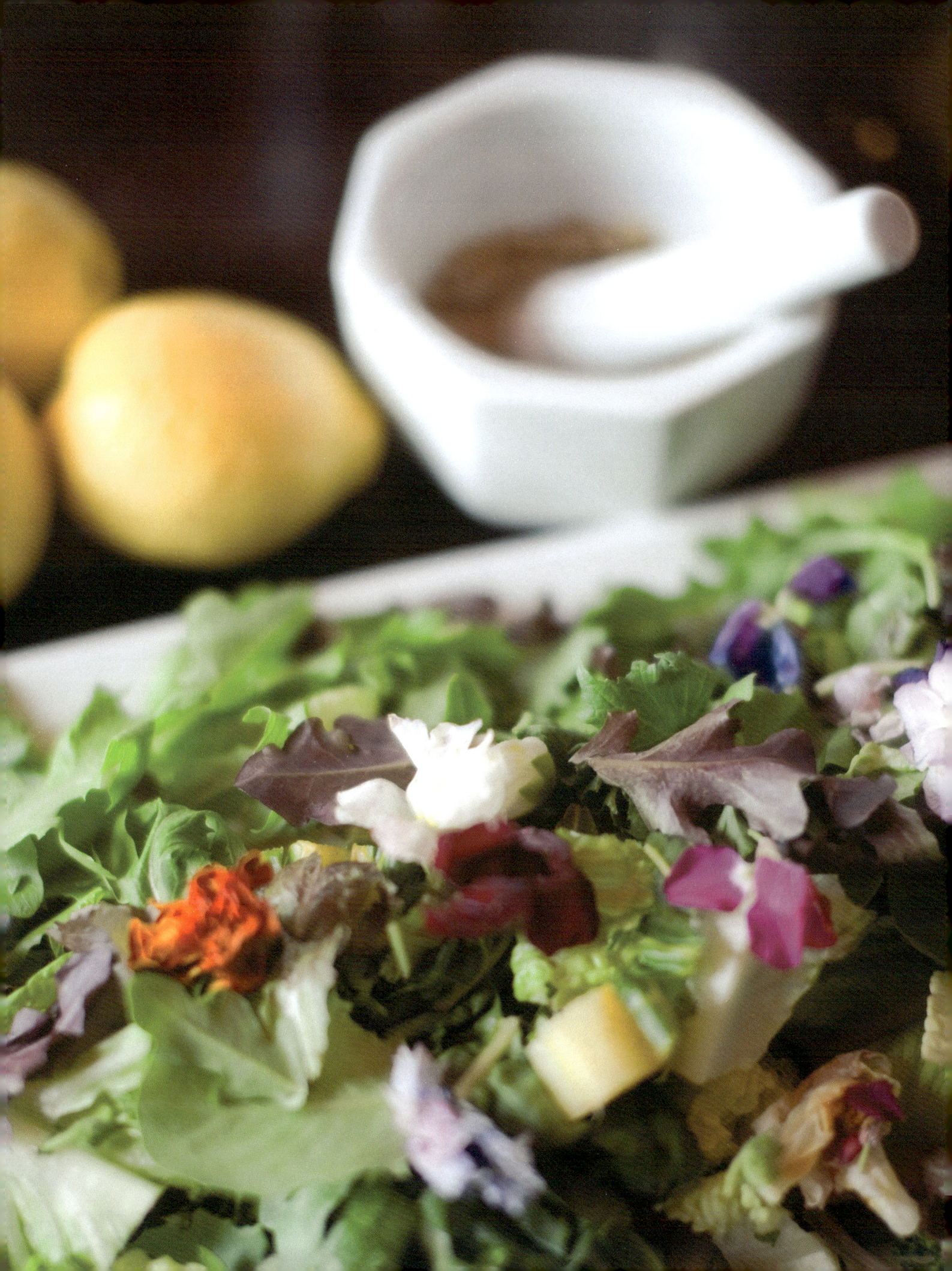

ODE TO AUTUMN SALAD & PAN DRIPPING DRESSING
serves 4

This autumn inspired salad will send wafts of comfort throughout your home and provide a rich, nourishing dish to your table. The fall season brings me a lot of bliss. I love the smells, the crispness in the air, and the overall assortment of marvelous foods to create. In addition, when it comes to vegetables and fruit, I believe the more the merrier!

3 tablespoons coconut oil (I have also used sesame oil)
1 large apple, cut into full moon circles, then quarter
1 sweet potato cut in half moon wedges
3 shallots, thinly slice
½ cup walnuts, chopped
1 tablespoon black sesame seeds
1 teaspoon freshly grated nutmeg
sea salt to taste
2 tablespoons pure maple syrup
6 cups mixed greens
½ teaspoon white pepper
Pan Dripping Dressing

Preheat oven to 375 °F.

Oil your roasting pan with coconut oil. Add apple, sweet potato, shallots, and walnuts. Sprinkle sesame seeds and freshly grated nutmeg over top. Sprinkle with a pinch of sea salt and maple syrup, and toss to coat.

Bake for about 25 minutes. Allow to cool.

On a serving platter, scatter your mixed greens. Spoon the roasted goodness onto the bed of greens. Drizzle with Pan Dripping Dressing.

PAN DRIPPING DRESSING

Add 1 ½ tablespoons organic apple cider vinegar to pan drippings left over from roasting. Whisk together and pour over top of salad. If needed, add more oil, sea salt, and pepper to taste.

Each of these will make well over a cup. Refrigerate and use within 2-3 days.

AIRMID'S HERBAL DRESSING:
1 garlic clove, minced, 1 tablespoon vegan mayo, pinch of raw cane sugar, 1 teaspoon fresh thyme, minced, 1 teaspoon fresh oregano, minced, 1 teaspoon fresh mint, minced, 1 teaspoon fresh basil, minced, 1 ½ teaspoon fresh squeezed lemon juice, 3 ¼ teaspoons balsamic vinegar, ¾ cup extra virgin olive oil, sea salt and fresh ground pepper to taste. Combine all the ingredients except the olive oil, salt and pepper. Slowly whisk in the oil until well blended. Season to taste with salt and pepper.

THE SUMMER SOLSTICE DRESSING:
1½ cups vegan mayo, ¾ extra virgin olive oil, ¼ brown rice vinegar, 1 tablespoon lemon juice, 3 tablespoons shallots, minced, 1 ½ teaspoon raw cane sugar, ¾ teaspoon sea salt, 1 garlic clove, minced. Combine all ingredients in a blender. Cover and process until smooth. Season with salt and pepper, if desired.

KIRA-KIRA DRESSING:
1 cup vegan mayo, ⅓ cup chives, chopped, 2 shallots, chopped, 1 clove garlic, peeled, 1 tablespoon brown rice vinegar, 1 teaspoon dill, chopped, 1 teaspoon raw cane sugar, 1 teaspoon Bragg's Liquid Aminos. Combine vegan mayo, chives, shallots, garlic, vinegar, dill, sugar, and Bragg's in a blender. Blend till smooth. Season with salt and pepper to taste.

THE JEWEL OF WINTER VINAIGRETTE:
¼ cup extra-virgin olive oil, 1 ½ tablespoons freshly squeezed orange juice, 3 tablespoons pomegranate juice, ½ tablespoons apple cider vinegar, ½ teaspoon sea salt, ¼ teaspoon freshly grated orange peel, pinch of cinnamon. Place all ingredients into a glass jar and shake well.

ANU'S VINAIGRETTE:
Roughly chop fresh herbs of choice (a handful or two will do depending on size of vinegar bottle) and about 2 cloves peeled garlic. Place into a large bottle and fill with vinegar. Allow to steep for about two weeks.

THE GYPSY'S DRESSING:
6 tablespoons lemon juice, 2 tablespoons sesame oil, 4 teaspoons brown rice syrup, 2 teaspoons grated lemon peel, 2 teaspoons fresh mint leaves, finely chopped. Combine ingredients and whisk well.

THE GEISHA'S VINAIGRETTE:
3 cloves garlic, minced, 2 ½ tablespoons fresh ginger, minced, ½ cup extra virgin olive oil, ¼ cup sesame oil, ⅓ cup rice vinegar, ¼ cup shoyu, 3 tablespoons agave, ¼ cup warm/hot water. Combine all ingredients in jar. Cover jar with lid and shake well. Chill and shake well before serving.

MONKS MARINADE:
1 tablespoon whole mustard seeds, ½ cup extra-virgin olive oil, ¼ brown rice vinegar, 3 tablespoons agave, ½ tablespoon Dijon mustard, 1 teaspoon dried rosemary, sea salt and ground pepper to taste. Toast mustard seeds in a dry skillet and cover. Sauté over medium-high heat. Once the seeds begin to pop, remove from heat. Combine the toasted seeds, oil, vinegar, agave, mustard, rosemary, salt, and pepper.

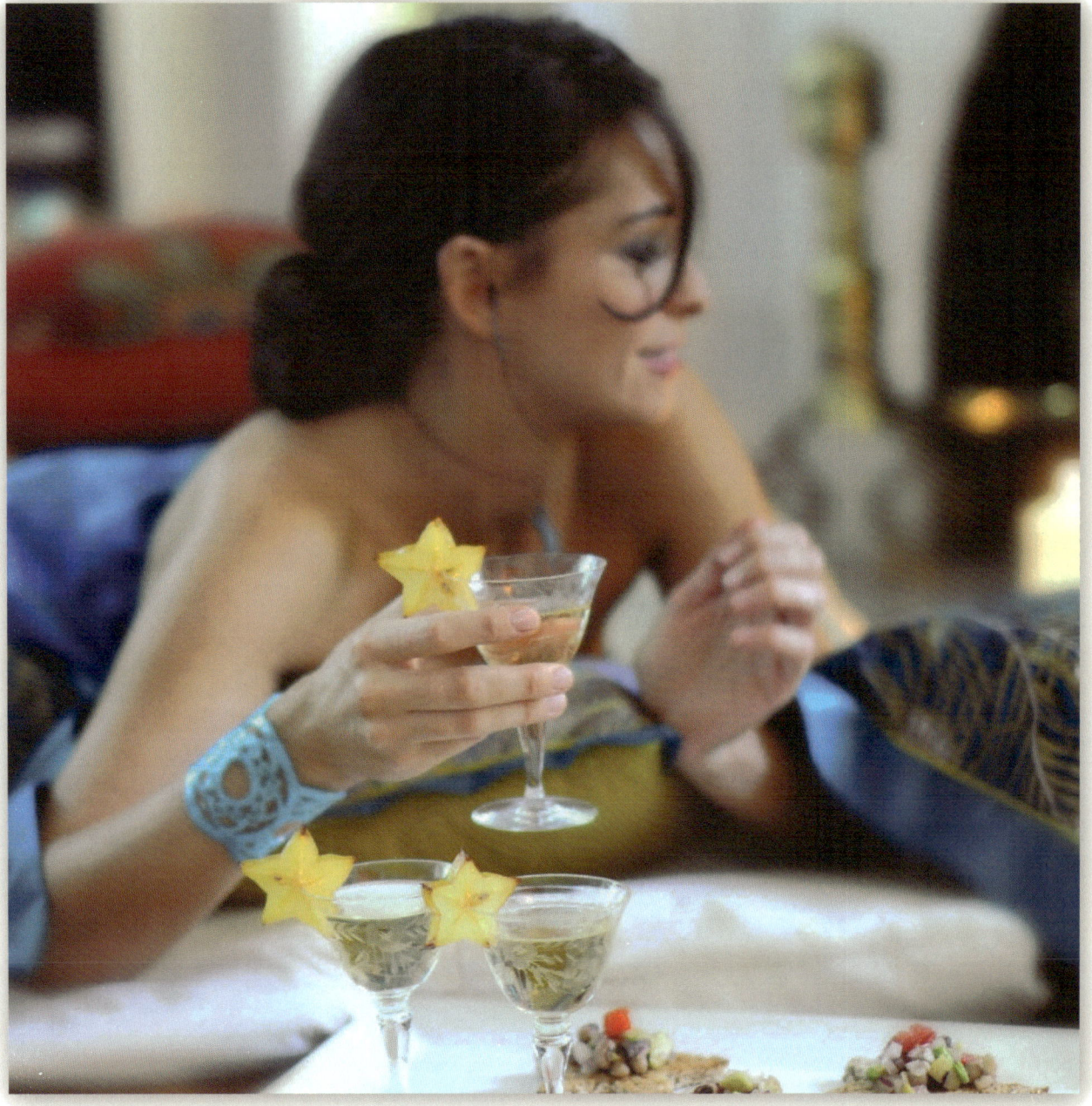

Musing No. 33

The universe is full of magical things just waiting for us to discover and unfold. Find ways to add layers of magical charms to your gatherings and embrace your artistic flare. This will offer a subtle nuance that is sure to not go unnoticed.

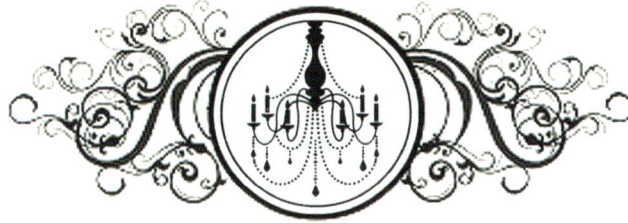

PETITE BITES

WITH A STASH OF HEALTHY RECIPES AND A CREATIVE IMAGINATION, A SIMPLE GATHERING WILL COME TOGETHER EFFORTLESSLY. WHAT IS PREPARED SOMETIMES IS SIMPLY BASED ON WHAT WE HAVE IN OUR PANTRY OR REFRIGERATOR. YOU KNOW THE SONG AND DANCE: SIMPLE, QUICK, HEALTHY, AND COLORFUL ARE MUST HAVES FOR CREATING A MEMORABLE, INTIMATE, NO-FUSS GET TOGETHER.

BRUSCHETTA CROWNED WITH CRUNCHY SPROUTS

serves 12

Eat things that make your eyes dance with a menagerie of colors! Find ways to bring your favorite vegetables into your next gathering. I love the basic purpose of the bruschetta and the sturdiness of the bread to hold some serious delicious ingredients.

4 medium tomatoes, chopped
4 - 5 basil leaves, chopped
12 slices whole wheat bread, sliced
3 cloves garlic, peeled and sliced
6 - 7 tablespoons extra virgin olive oil
3 avocados, peeled, seeded and mashed
2 tablespoons lime juice
sea salt and fresh ground pepper to taste
1 cup pine nuts, toasted
1 cup spicy sprouts

Place chopped tomatoes in a small bowl, and season with salt and pepper. Stir in the basil. Allow to set for 15 minutes.

Broil or toast the bread until crispy on both sides. Cut garlic in half and rub on one side of each piece of toast. Arrange garlic-rubbed toast onto a platter, and sprinkle with olive oil.

Mash the avocado in small bowl with a fork until creamy. Add lime juice and mix well. Spoon the avocado mix onto the top of each bruschetta. Spoon the chopped tomato mixture on each one.

Sprinkle each with toasted pine nuts. Top with crunchy sprouts.

Drizzle the platter with extra virgin olive oil, and season with salt and pepper.

Musing No. 34

Mix rustic and earthy elements with thrift store crystal like sea shells, vines, and herbs. Scatter them about to create a centerpiece for your buffet or bar. Display your finest thrift store crystal filled to the rim with creative concoctions.

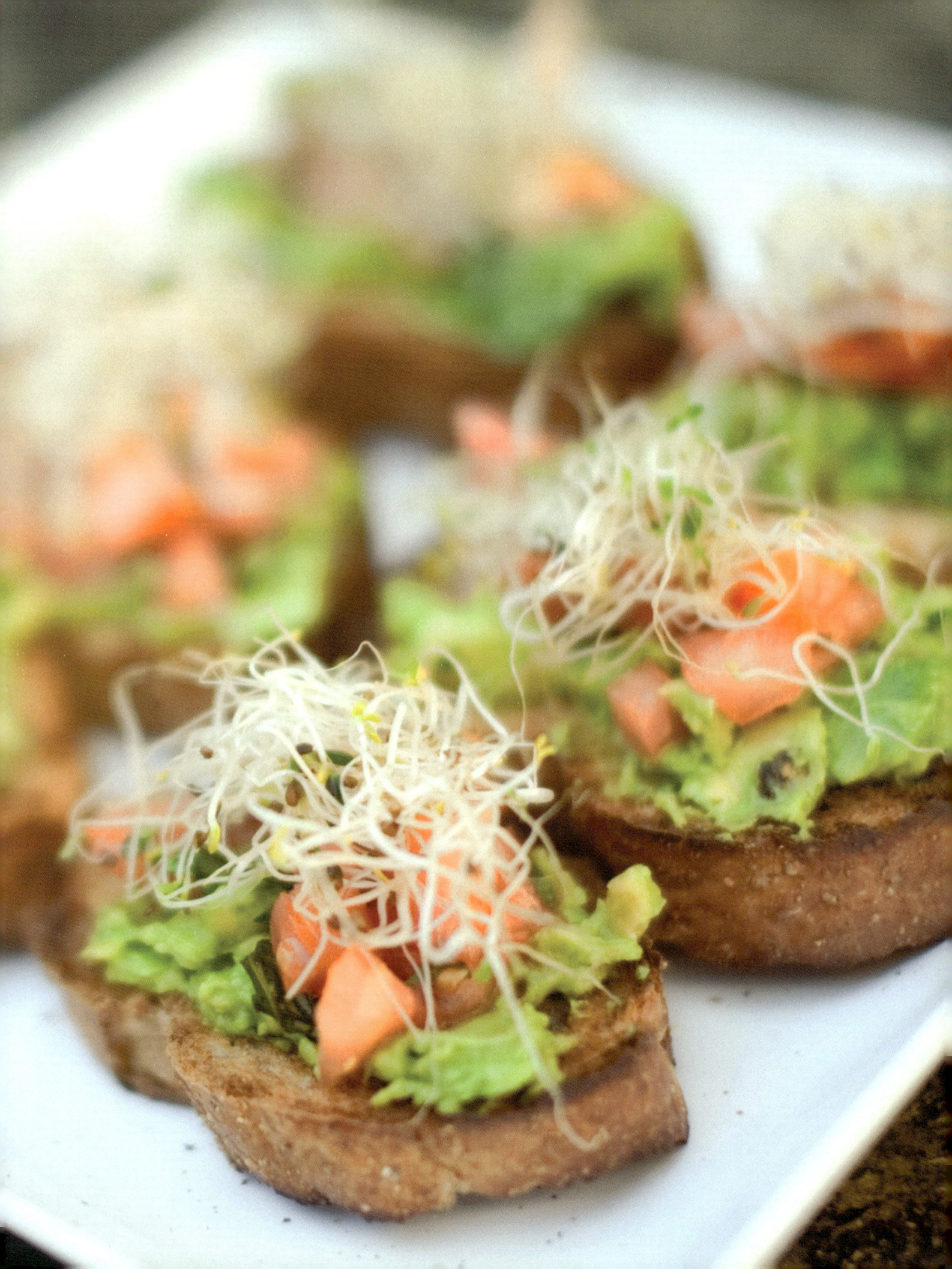

GYPSY MOON PATE WITH PITA POINTS
serves 12

This enchanting mix of spices, molasses, and vegetables creates an exotic Moroccan gypsy inspired creation. I have many simple yet sophisticated pates and dips, but this one is just one of my favorites. It is easy to make and has those old-world flavors layered throughout that I just crave. If the pomegranate molasses is hard to find, try with black strap molasses.

¾ cup walnuts, lightly toasted
2 ½ large red bell peppers, roasted, peeled and seeded
1 fresh red chili pepper, roasted, peeled and seeded
2 scallions, chopped
½ cup stone ground whole wheat crackers, crumbled
1 tablespoon lemon juice, fresh squeezed
1 ½ tablespoons pomegranate molasses or black strap molasses
⅓ tablespoon ground cumin
½ teaspoon turbinado sugar
sea salt to taste
1 ½ tablespoons extra virgin olive oil, a bit more for garnish
2 tablespoons pine nuts, toasted

In a food processor, finely chop walnuts. Add the peppers, chili pepper, scallions, crackers, juice, molasses, cumin, sugar, and salt. When mix is smooth, slowly pour in the oil. Sample the flavors; add more lemon juice, molasses, or salt as needed.

This pate is best if you can allow the flavors to meld overnight. Before serving, drizzle top with some extra oil, add a pinch or two of cumin, and sprinkle with toasted pine nuts.

PITA POINTS

3 tablespoons olive oil
2 garlic cloves, minced
¼ teaspoon oregano
¼ teaspoon sea salt
fresh ground pepper to taste (optional)
2 regular sized pita pockets

Preheat oven to 375 °F.

In a small bowl, mix olive oil, garlic, oregano, salt, and pepper. Using kitchen scissors, cut pita pockets into 4 even wedges. Slice wedges in half, and then slice each half once more to make 16 wedges. Cut along the curved outer edge to separate the two sides of the pita. Brush both sides of wedges with olive oil mixture. Coat well.

Bake for about 10 minutes or until golden brown.

SHEBAT'S HUMMUS & CRUDITE PLATTER
Serves 4 - 6

Creating a memorable gathering that is intimate, free-spirited, and full of endless, fascinating conversations is quite simple. As the host, enjoying yourself is a key element. No need to overcomplicate things by spending too much time stressing out over what to serve or spending too much money on the food. Instead, focus on creating an ambiance that is stress-free. Life is just too short to not enjoy the moment. This is one of those quickie appetizers that I can whip up blindfolded with one hand tied behind my back. It's something that everyone is tempted to swoop into, dip, and crunch on.

SHEBAT'S HUMMUS

2 tablespoons extra-virgin olive oil
juice of 1 lemon
2 teaspoons ground curry
2 garlic cloves, peeled
¼ cup tahini
1 ½ cups garbanzo beans, pre-cooked
dash paprika (optional)

Place oil, juice, curry, garlic, tahini and garbanzo beans into blender and blend until smooth. Sprinkle with paprika (optional).

CRUDITÉ

With your crudité platter, be mindful of the number of guests. This will determine your amounts. Usually, I will just grab handfuls of each veggie and place them into glass containers or just arrange on a platter.

Belgian endive, root ends removed and leaves separated
whole snap peas
carrots, scraped and cut into 3-by-¼ inch strips
fennel, trimmed and cut into strips
whole button mushrooms
jicama, peeled and cut into 3-by-¼ inch strips
zucchini, cut into 3-by-¼ inch strips

Wash and prepare your veggies and arrange them decoratively on platter. Serve with hummus for dipping.

Musing No. 36
For the bling factor at your next gathering, simply light a plethora of candles.

MON COCO BITES & DIP
serves 6 - 8

I am smitten by the coconut not only for its medicinal purposes but for its slightly sweet milk, rich meat, and its ability to offer itself for many uses. This botanical nut is revered in many rituals across the globe to ensure blessings and is a symbol of auspiciousness.

COCONUT BITES

1 pound organic tempeh, plain
½ cup coconut milk
1 tablespoons lime juice
½ cup oat flour
½ cup unsweetened coconut flakes
½ cup coconut oil
sea salt and fresh ground pepper to taste

Line a plate with a clean kitchen towel.

Cut tempeh into 1-inch squares.

In a small bowl, mix together the coconut milk, lime juice, flour, and coconut flakes.

In a frying pan, heat the coconut oil over high heat. Coat each tempeh square with the flour mixture. Fry until golden brown on both sides. Transfer to kitchen towel to drain. Sprinkle with salt and pepper.

DIP

½ cup vegan mayo
3 scallions, finely chopped
2 garlic cloves, minced
1 handful fresh cilantro, finely chopped
1 6-oz can pureed chipotle chili, drained

In a small bowl, add vegan mayo, scallions, garlic, cilantro, and chipotle chili. Mix well, and chill for about 30 minutes.

Place Coconut Bites on serving platter, and place dip into a ramekin.

Musing No. 37
In Sanskrit, the coconut palm is known as kalpa vriksha...tree which gives all that is necessary for living.

VOODOO STUFFED CAPS

serves 12

This recipe is an authentic blend of Middle Eastern spices paired with a mushroom and what a marvelous container to hold such divine flavors. I do love a delicious accident. I was making my usual Chickpea Pate to spread on croquettes one evening for an impromptu gathering and realized that I had no bread! I was going to make mushroom caps anyway, so instead of pulling together my usual mushroom stuffing, I used what I had already prepared. It turned out to be a wonderful contrast of flavors. Cheers to the many "accidents" in life.

CHICKPEA MIXTURE

2 14-ounce cans chickpeas, rinsed and drained
6 - 8 sun-dried tomatoes packed in oil, drained
2 shallots, chopped
¼ cup extra virgin olive oil
2 teaspoon sumac
1 teaspoon ground coriander
1 teaspoon ground cumin
3 cloves garlic, peeled
12 button mushroom caps, hollowed out
½ teaspoon white pepper
1 teaspoon sea salt

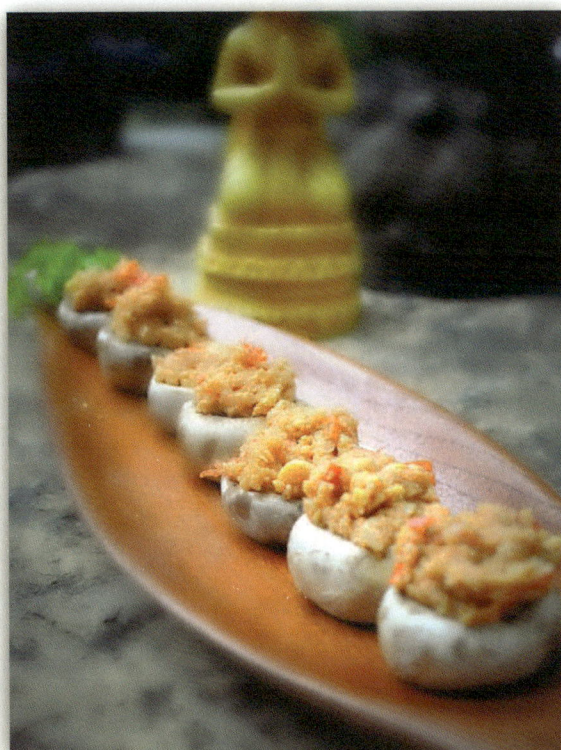

Preheat oven to 375 °F.

In a food processor, add chickpeas, tomatoes, and shallots. Process until smooth. Add in the oil, and blend. Add in sumac, coriander, cumin, and garlic, and puree to smooth.

Remove stems from mushrooms. Oil a baking dish and place mushrooms smooth side down. Sprinkle with sea salt and pepper. Bake for about 20 minutes. When cooled, spoon chickpea mixture into each mushroom cap.

Sprinkle with sea salt to taste, and garnish by dusting with cumin and fresh parsley.

AVOCADO CAVIAR ON STARS
WITH A DASH OF KIRA-KIRA DRESSING
serves 12

Kira is an ancient name. Its Sanskrit meaning is "beam of light." In Japanese, the term Kira kira means "glittery and sparkly." This was the inspiration to serve the bean salad or "caviar" on top of starry toast points! Of course, the stars are just for the whim and fancy of it; toast points are perfectly fine.

2 cups black-eyed peas, pre-cooked
2 tomatoes, finely diced
1 can green chilies, drained and diced
2 avocados, peeled, pitted and diced
½ red onion, diced
⅓ cup Kira-Kira Dressing (page 64)
3 tablespoons fresh squeezed lime juice
½ teaspoon sea salt
12 whole grain bread slices, cut with star-shaped cookie cutter and toasted

In a large bowl, mix together black-eyed peas, tomatoes, chilies, avocados, red onion, Kira-Kira Dressing, lime juice, and salt. Cover and chill.

Toast star-shaped bread. Allow bread to cool. Top each star with caviar.

Musing No. 38

Stars are a muse to Mother Earth. The nearest star to our planet is the Sun. This luminous ornament that adorns our sky provides most of our planet's energy.

Musing No. 39

Light incense sticks to create a permeating waft of exotic ambiance for your gathering.

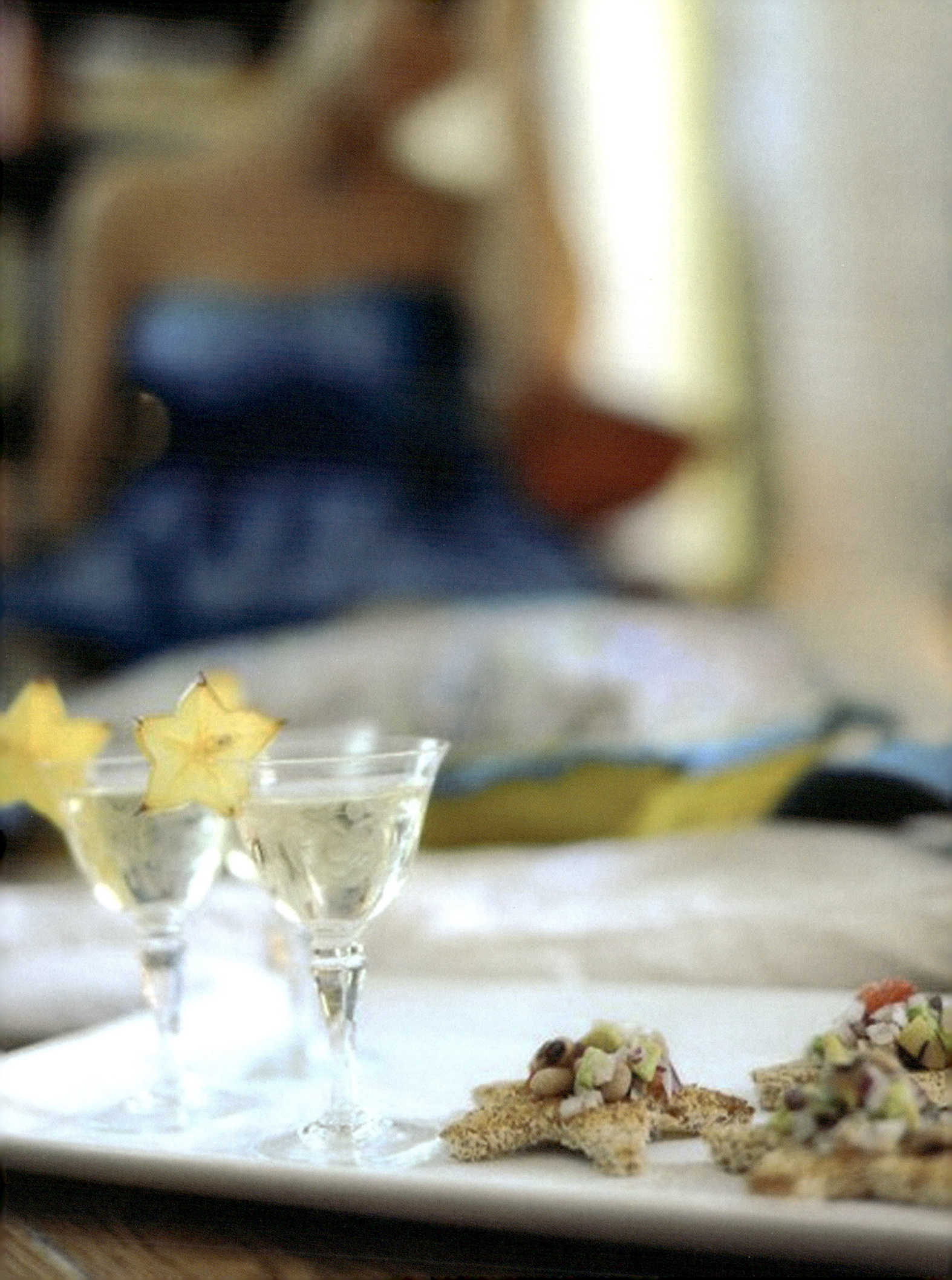

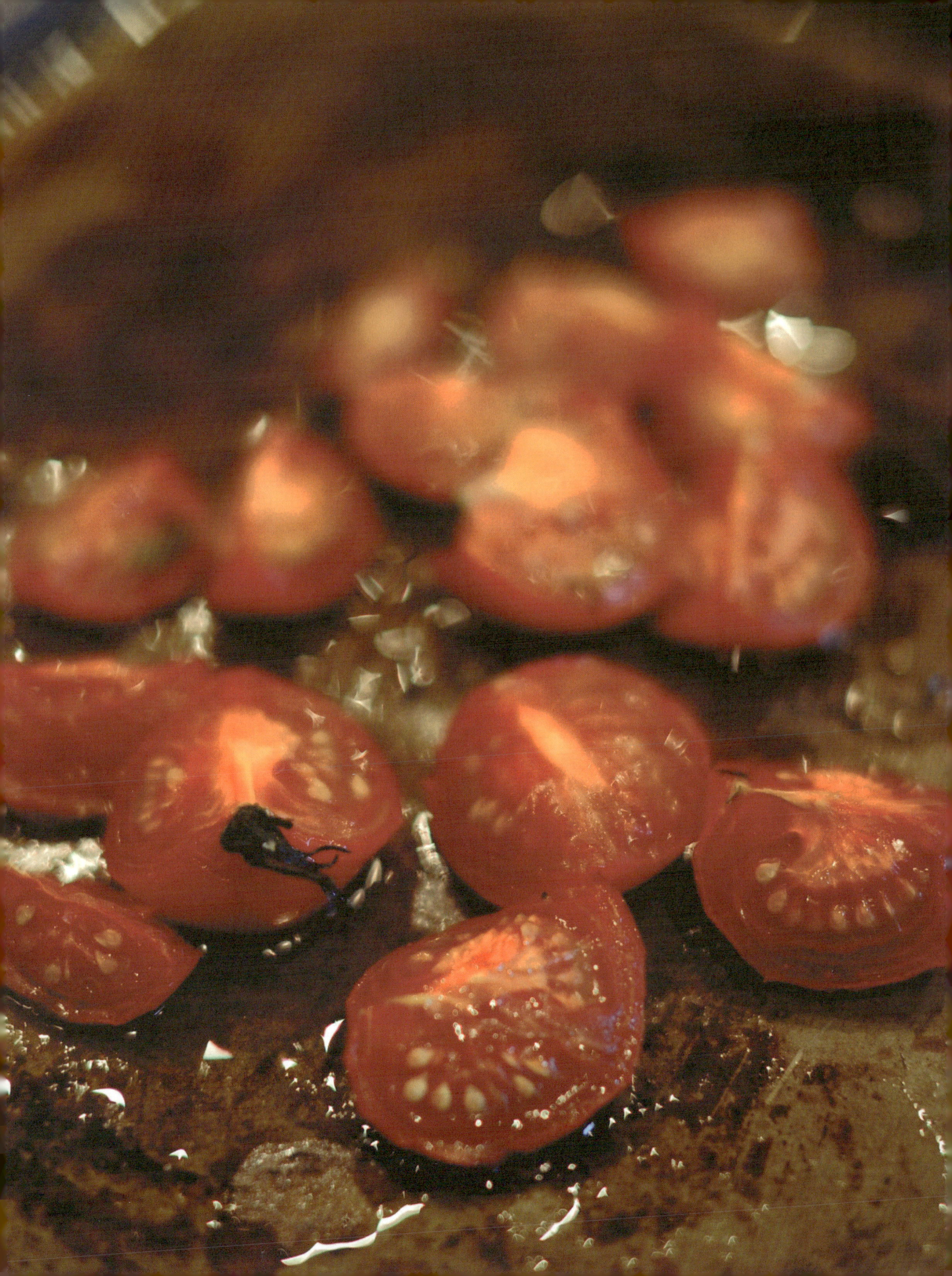

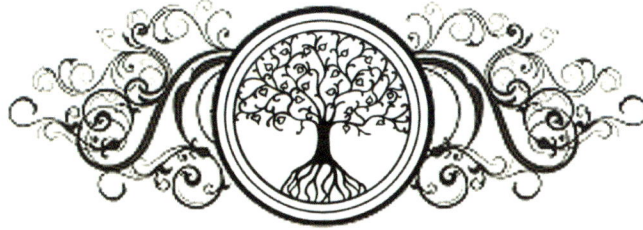

SIDES

Spoil yourself, your family, or someone you adore and indulge in tantalizing side dishes that create a dinner worth lingering over. Light up some candles, put on some music, and enjoy preparing your culinary creations to offer on your table this eve.

BRUSSELS SPROUTS AND MUSTARD BUTTER
serves 6

Cultivated in ancient Rome, the Brussels sprout became quite popular and spread into the southern Netherlands and into parts of Northern Europe. This well traveled sprout offers a potent mix of healing properties. A chemical called indole-3-carbinol, found in this enchanted food, helps repair DNA in cells and is said to block the growth of cancer cells. So much goodness offered from the plant world. I love earthy flavors so, to me, a Brussels sprout is just divine on its own, but when paired with a bold mustard, it evolves into a somewhat of a serendipitous union.

1 pound Brussels sprouts
1 ½ teaspoons tarragon vinegar
1 clove garlic, minced
1 ½ tablespoons whole grain Dijon mustard
6 - 8 tablespoons vegan butter, room temperature
2 small shallots, minced
2 tablespoons parsley, finely chopped
1 teaspoon sea salt
1 teaspoon ground pepper
½ teaspoon caraway seeds, bruised in mortar

In a large pot, bring about 3 - 4 cups of water to a boil.

Slice sprouts in half lengthwise. Sprinkle water with sea salt and add sprouts. Cook for about 6 minutes.

MUSTARD BUTTER

Drain and place sprouts into a serving dish. Sprinkle with tarragon vinegar and toss to coat. In a separate bowl, whisk together garlic, mustard, vegan butter, shallots, and parsley. Pour over top of Brussels sprouts, coating well. Season with sea salt, pepper, and caraway seeds. "In a separate bowl, whisk together garlic, mustard, vegan butter, shallots, and parsley.

Musing No. 40
I always find dinner to be a magical time to unwind from the day. Setting a mood as if it were already the weekend always works like a charm.

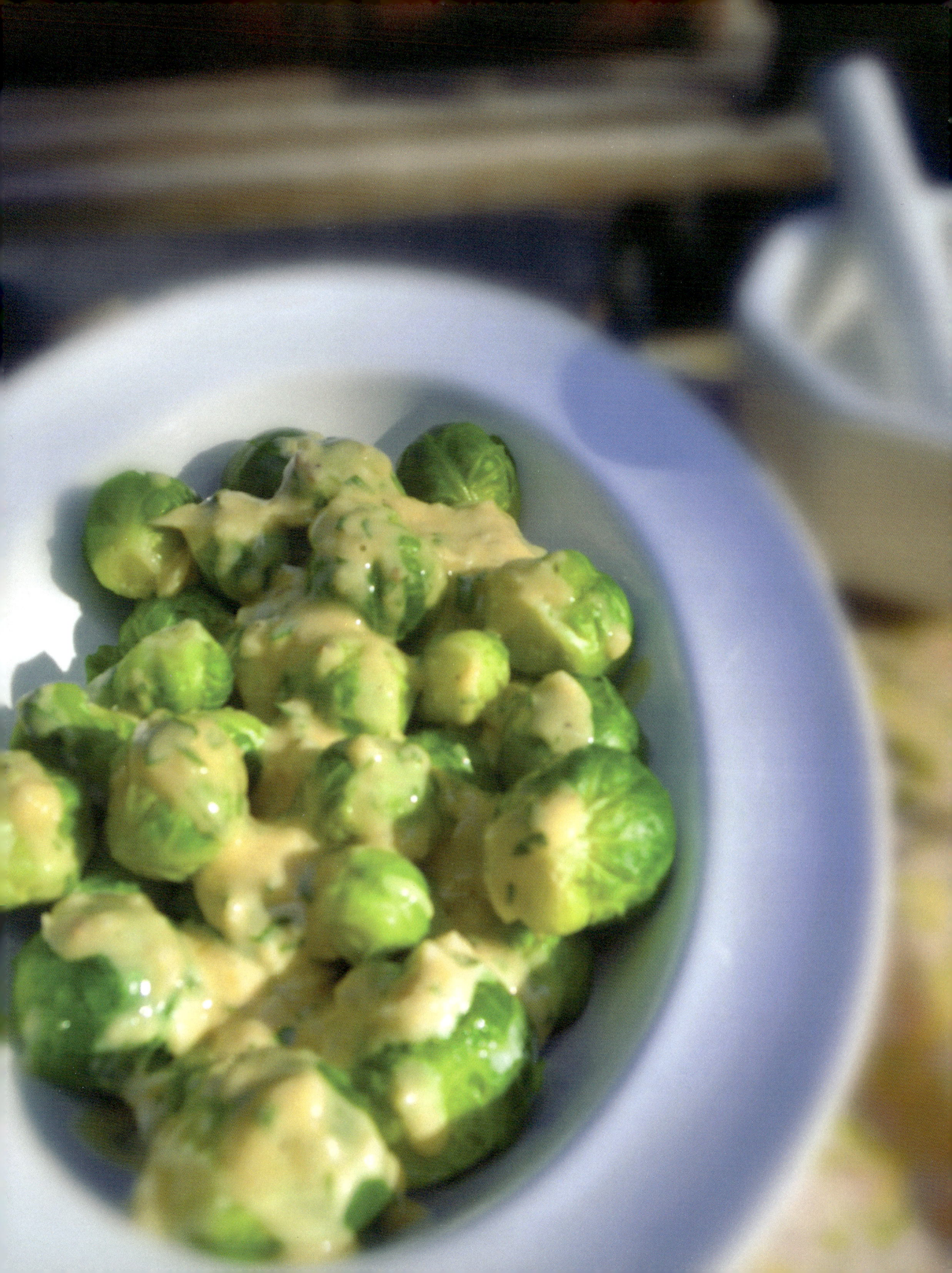

BRAISED LENTILS SCENTED WITH AROMATICS

serves 6 - 8

I love the soft texture of lentils. They are the perfect companion for aromatics. This dish is a comfort food for me, dressed with distinctive flavors of aromatics. This just proves how easily a legume goes from understated to uniquely elegant.

2 ⅓ cups lentils
5 - 6 tablespoons extra virgin olive oil
1 small onion, finely chopped
2 cloves garlic, minced
1 carrot, finely chopped
2 celery stalks, finely chopped
1 dried red chili, chopped
½ teaspoon turmeric
1 ¼ cups red wine
2 bay leaves
3 ½ cups veggie stock
sea salt and fresh ground pepper to taste
1 teaspoon mustard seeds
⅓ cup parsley, chopped

Wash the lentils in a few changes of water.

In a skillet, drizzle with olive oil over medium high heat and sauté the onion, garlic, carrot, celery, and chili for about a minute. Set aside for a bit.

In a separate pot drizzled with a bit of olive oil, add lentils, turmeric, red wine, bay leaves, and veggie stock. Bring to a boil and simmer; cover for about 30 minutes or just until tender. Season with salt and pepper to taste.

Re-heat skillet of vegetables and add in mustard seeds and sauté over high heat until seeds begin to turn grayish, about a minute.

Pour over lentils, mix well, and transfer to a serving platter and top with fresh parsley.

Musing No. 41

Baking soda is an eco-friendly way to clean pots & pans.

ROASTED SQUASH WITH INDIAN SPICES
serves 6 - 8

I am overcome by the warmth and richness this dish offers. The fragrances alone will envelope your senses. There is a brilliance of spices that is truly magical. This is one of my favorites for the holiday seasons. It's sort of my fantasy dish.

2 ½ to 3 pounds acorn squash
⅓ cup extra virgin olive oil
2 teaspoons brown rice syrup

Preheat oven to 375 °F.

Cut squash in half and remove seeds. Brush well with olive oil and place the cut-sides down on a baking sheet. Pour about ½ inch water and bake until tender, about 25 minutes.

Remove from oven and drizzle with brown rice syrup. Sprinkle the Indian Spiced Sea Salt and serve.

INDIAN SPICED SEA SALT

2 tablespoons sesame seeds
2 tablespoons coriander seeds
1 ½ tablespoons cumin seeds
2 tablespoons sea salt
⅓ teaspoon cayenne pepper

Toast sesame, coriander, and cumin seeds in a dry skillet over medium heat, until fragrant. Allow to cool.

In a mortar and pestle, grind toasted ingredients with sea salt and cayenne pepper until fine.

Sprinkle overtop roasted squash.

Musing No. 42

Light up some candles. Play some music. Play a game of cards or chess. Let your dinner time amuse you.

SAVORY DINNER MUFFINS
serves 15

I have this thing for comfort foods, ones that are simple, earthy, and healthy. Savory muffins are just one of those that you can keep simple or dress up with glorious fixings such as fancy herb butter, pepper gravy, or just a pat of vegan butter. It's just another spirited goody to bring to the "altar" (table). The reason for the serving size in this particular recipe is because these are so easy to freeze and warm when needed. I have found that I like the fluffiness of these, so I use them as biscuits.

SAVORY DINNER MUFFINS

1 cup chickpea flour
3 cups white whole wheat pastry flour
3 teaspoons cumin
3 teaspoons garam masala
2 teaspoons red pepper flakes
2 scallions, chopped finely
2 teaspoons baking powder, aluminum free
1 teaspoon baking soda
2 teaspoons sea salt
½ tablespoon tahini
¼ cup toasted sesame oil
3 ½ teaspoons agave nectar
2 ½ cups almond milk, plain

Preheat oven to 350 °F.

Line muffin tins, or wipe down with oil.

In a large bowl, combine the chickpea and pastry flour, cumin, garam masala, red pepper flakes, scallions, baking powder, baking soda, and salt.

In a separate bowl, mix together the tahini, oil, agave, and milk. Fold the wet ingredients into the dry mix. Do not over-mix. Spoon batter equally among the muffin cups.

Bake for about 15 minutes, or until fork inserted comes out clean. Spread each savory dinner muffin with Persillade Butter. (page 82)

Musing No. 43

Don't always use the same oil. Use coconut oil, sesame oil, almond oil, or the good old stand by extra virgin olive oil.

SWEETLY SPICED CORNBREAD
serves 12

Ahh... cornbread and soup. Now that's a romance worthy of a novel. The two were simply meant to be. Together they offer such warm, rustic goodness (not to mention slathering up a sliver of cornbread fresh from the oven with vegan butter). I love the sweetness the maple syrup brings for further enhancement to the earthiness of this cornbread.

½ cup wheat pastry flour
1 ½ cups cornmeal
1 teaspoon baking soda
½ teaspoon sea salt
¼ teaspoon ground nutmeg
¼ teaspoon ground cardamom
¼ cup safflower oil, plus extra for pan
1 cup pure maple syrup
1 ½ cups hemp milk, plain

Preheat oven to 400 °F.

Drizzle oil into cast iron cornbread pan and heat for 5 minutes in preheated oven.

In a mixing bowl, combine flour, cornmeal, baking soda, salt, nutmeg, and cardamom. In a separate bowl, combine oil, syrup, and milk together and whisk.

Pour half of milk mixture into dry ingredients; slowly adding milk to dry. Stir just until moist. If more milk is needed to thin out mixture, then add the remaining milk mixture.

Pull cast iron pan from oven, and carefully pour cornbread mixture into hot oil. Spread with plain vegan butter or some Persillade Butter.

Bake for 25 minutes.

PERSILLADE BUTTER

This really is just a fancy and quick butter. Persillade is often described in recipes as one clove of garlic to a bunch of parsley, chopped well, and scattered over a dish. This is a no-fuss way to serve up just a layer of flavor to melt onto Savory Dinner Muffins. Remember the "no rules" rule, so always use your creativity with these, and add in your herb of choice. That is half the fun of being a fearless vegan kitchen cook.

½ cup vegan margarine
1 clove garlic, peeled and chopped
1 small handful of parsley, chopped

Mix well in a small bowl. Crown tops of muffins, cornbread, and veggie side dishes with your fancy butter!

KALE, BEANS, AND CURRY SCENTED HERB SAUCE
serves 4 - 6

I would rather have kale on my table than fine china, and kale we have. I find that the charm of the kale is the health if offers. As for our thrift store china, well, that's its charm! It is well-traveled like a gypsy!

1 ½ tablespoons extra virgin olive oil
2 pounds kale, stems removed
3 small shallots, minced
2 garlic cloves, minced
½ cup white wine
2 cups cannelloni, pre-cooked

Simmer the kale in salted water until tender, about 5 minutes. Drain and chop leaves.

In a skillet, drizzle oil and sauté the shallots and garlic for about 2 minutes. Add the wine, and cook until it is reduced.

Add the beans, kale, and a few splashes of leftover cooking water, and heat through. Place mix into a serving bowl.

CURRY SCENTED HERB SAUCE

2 cups vegetable stock
4 tablespoons coconut butter
2 tablespoons thyme, rough chopped
2 tablespoons marjoram, rough chopped
2 ½ teaspoons curry powder
2 teaspoons sea salt
1 teaspoon grated lemon zest

In a small sauce pan, heat veggie stock and coconut butter. Sprinkle in thyme, marjoram, curry powder, sea salt, and lemon zest. Mix well and ladle over top of kale and white bean mixture. Sprinkle with sea salt and fresh ground pepper if desired.

Musing No. 44
Knowing where your food comes from is invaluable.

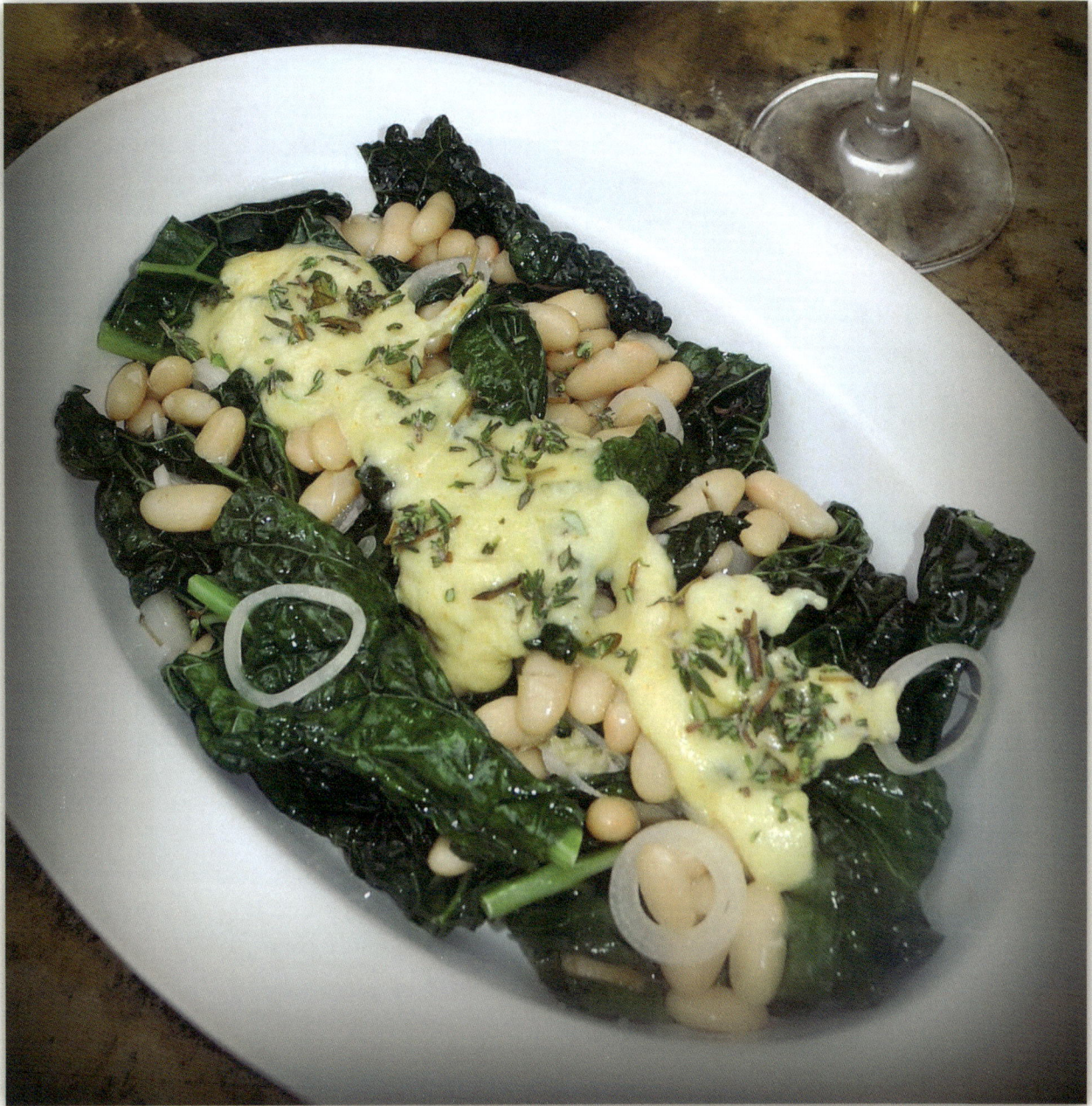

Musing No. 45

Linger longer at dinner.

CHAMPAGNE RISOTTO WITH
ROSEMARY & APPLES
serves 4

Just as rosemary is known as the herb of remembrance, this one dish wonder will be remembered long after the dinner hours. My goal with this recipe was to pleasantly enhance this already-layered dish with a nip of sparkling champagne. The combination for me made pure decadence.

3 tablespoons extra virgin olive oil
2 shallots, minced
1 celery stalk, finely chopped
2 cloves garlic, minced
1 cup Arborio rice (risotto rice)
5 cups vegetable broth
1 ½ cups dry champagne (you can also substitute the champagne with a white table wine if need be)
sea salt and fresh ground pepper to taste
½ cup apples, diced
¼ cup fresh rosemary, finely chopped
2 teaspoons fresh parsley, finely chopped

Sauté the shallots, celery and garlic in olive oil for 3 - 5 minutes or until soft. Add the risotto rice and cook, stirring constantly to avoid burning. Allow to cook for about 2 - 3 minutes or just until rice starts to brown. Add 1 cup vegetable broth and stir well to combine. Pour in champagne and stir. Add a dash of sea salt and pepper.

When most of the liquid has been absorbed, add in more broth a little at a time along with the apples, rosemary and parsley. The rice should be done in about 15 - 20 minutes. If the rice has absorbed all the stock and still needs further cooking, add a bit more water or broth.

Season generously with ground white pepper.

Musing No. 46
Organic farming shows respect for mother earth and the laws of nature.

STEAMED ARTICHOKES
serves 6

The ancients favored artichokes and considered them one of the greatest tokens of health from Mother Earth. The nutrient-rich flowering plant offers the most important minerals like chromium, potassium, iron, magnesium, calcium, and phosphorus. When these mossy-colored gems flower, they become an invitation to peel, saturate with seasonings, and indulge in the gifts of these spirited flower buds.

6 medium sized artichokes
2 lemons, halved
1 bay leaf
2 cloves garlic, peeled
5 tablespoons vegan butter
1 teaspoon sea salt
½ teaspoon cumin
1 cup whole wheat crackers, crumbled

Cut ½ inch from top of each artichoke. Remove the bottom leaves. Use kitchen scissors to cut about ½ inch off of the leaf tips. Place all prepared artichokes on cutting board and squeeze some lemon juice over top of each.

Fill a large pot with about 4 inches of water; add bay leaf and cloves of garlic. Squeeze the remaining lemon juice into water. Set artichokes, top down, in pot and bring to a boil. Reduce to medium heat and steam artichokes. Cover and steam for 40 - 45 minutes or until leaf is easy to pull away.

In a skillet, heat vegan butter on low and add in salt, cumin, and crumbled crackers.

Arrange artichokes on platter. Pour mix over top of each artichoke. This buttery mixture will fall into the open, flowered leaves, leaving you with a hearty, savory bite.

Drizzle each artichoke with Garlic Sauce. Sprinkle with sea salt and pepper to taste.

Musing No. 47

The "artichoke capital of the world," California, crowned Marilyn Monroe an "artichoke queen" in 1947. She inspired others to indulge in the benefits of this divine gem.

MARINATED RICE
serves 6 - 8

Consider elements that will add details of texture and color to your dishes. Remember, life is art and so are your dishes. Pick your favorite ingredients and discover a way to create an intriguing, conversational dish for your next gathering.

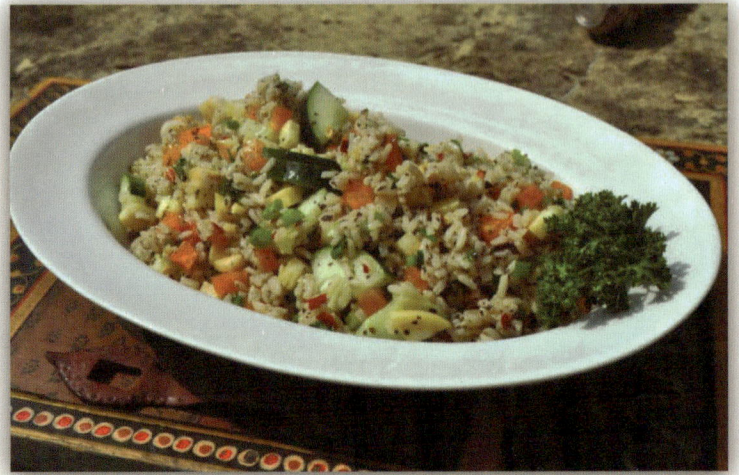

2 cups brown rice
2 ½ cups cherry tomatoes, chopped
4 scallions, chopped
1 stalk celery, diced
1 orange bell pepper, diced
1 cucumber, quartered and diced
1 ½ cups black eyed peas
½ cup sesame seeds, toasted
sea salt and fresh ground pepper to taste

Bring rice to a boil in covered saucepan. Reduce heat and simmer for about 20 minutes or until rice is tender. Fluff with fork and allow to cool.

Transfer to a large bowl and add in tomatoes, scallions, celery, orange bell pepper, cucumber, and black eyed peas. Mix well.

Pour Marinade overtop and stir well. Sprinkle with toasted sesame seeds, sea salt and pepper to taste.

MARINADE

½ cup sesame oil
¼ cup organic apple cider vinegar
2 tablespoons dried basil
½ cup fresh parsley
2 tablespoons red pepper flakes
1 tablespoon sea salt
fresh ground pepper to taste (optional)

In a small mixing bowl, whisk together all ingredients. Stir well and refrigerate until ready to pour over top of rice.

HERBED WEDGES & SPICY SAUCE
serves 6

I do hope you love homemade French fries as much as I do! My family loves them, my kids love them, and they're a classic treat that I am quite smitten by. This is one of those rituals that must always be served alongside our "meatless" burgers. They're even used sometimes as an appetizer for casual entertaining. It's so entirely easy. One has to love a recipe that only calls for a few simple ingredients. Don't forget to pair these deeply rooted veggies with fresh herbs for a hypnotic courtship.

4 tablespoons extra virgin olive oil
3 - 4 pounds potatoes, washed and peeled
1 tablespoon fresh rosemary, minced
1 tablespoon fresh thyme, minced
2 tablespoons fresh parsley, minced
sea salt and fresh ground pepper to taste

Preheat oven to 350 °F.

Wipe baking sheet with olive oil until thoroughly coated.

Cut the potatoes into wedge shapes. Toss the potato wedges, rosemary, thyme, and parsley in a bowl.

Pour herbed wedges onto baking sheet and sprinkle with sea salt and pepper to taste.

Bake for 25 minutes or until golden brown.

SPICY SAUCE

1 cup vegan mayo
⅓ cup fresh cilantro
2 tablespoons garlic, minced
4 scallions, finely chopped
1 tablespoon jalapeno, minced
1 tablespoon fresh lime juice
1 tablespoon sea salt
freshly ground white pepper

In small bowl, mix mayo, cilantro, garlic, scallions, jalapeno, lime juice, and salt. Sprinkle with fresh pepper and leftover cilantro.

Arrange wedges onto a serving dish. Pour spicy sauce over top or simply place sauce into a ramekin and serve for dipping.

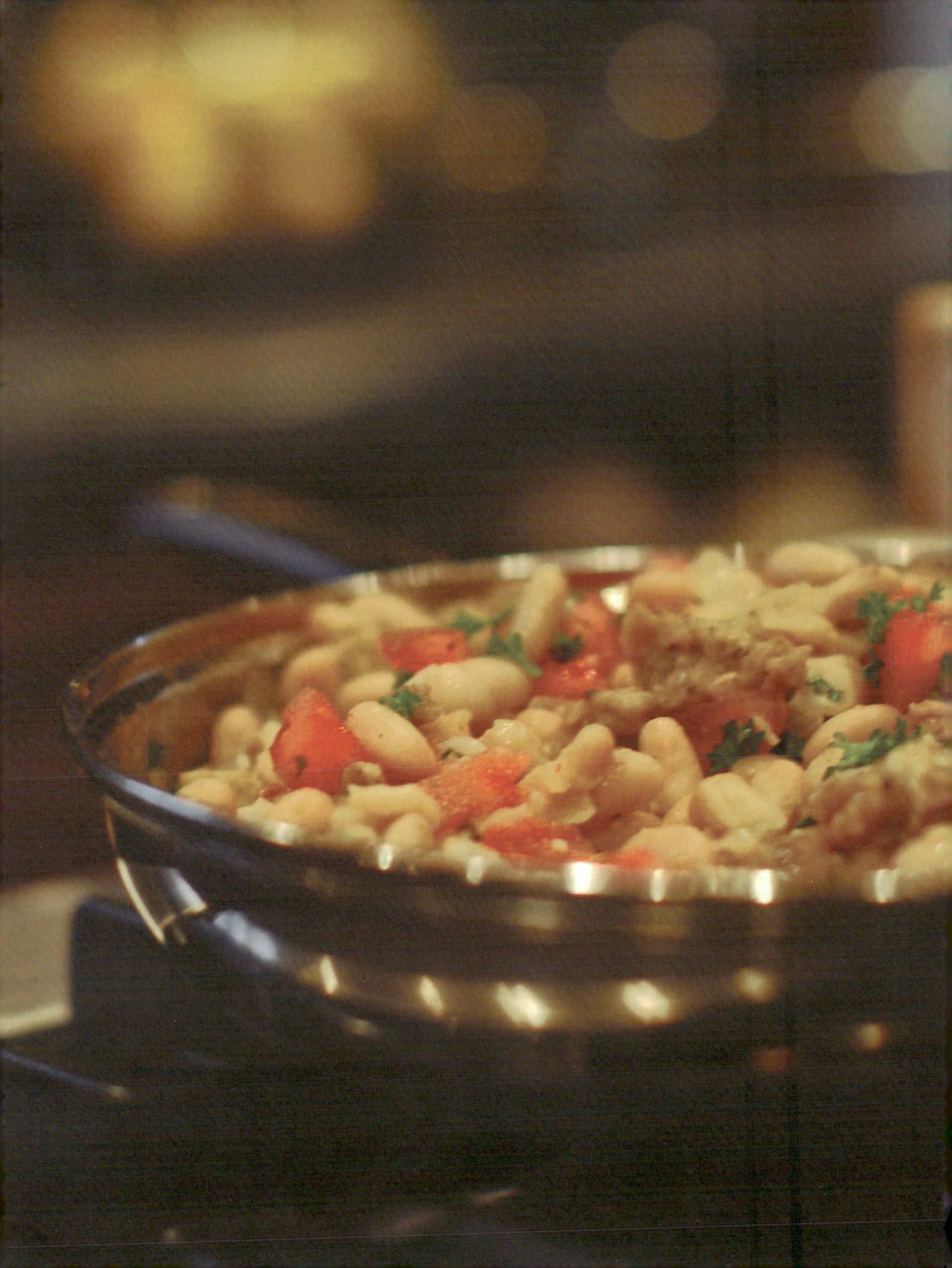

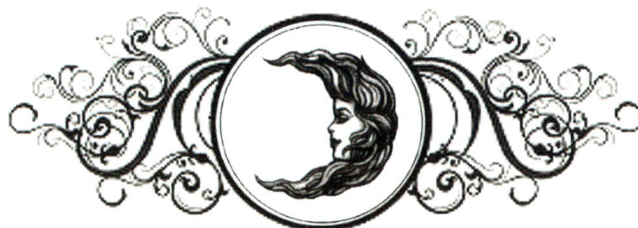

DINNERS

I can tell you, without hesitation, I am a believer that the kitchen is the soul of the home. It's that one place where wafts of comfort come from, where spirited conversations are had, and swoon-worthy dinners are created.

SLOPPY VEGAN BURGERS

serves 6 - 8

The Incas endearingly named quinoa "the mother of all grains" and native Peruvians refer to it as vegetable caviar. It was believed that this pseudo-grain contained magical properties and was consumed sometimes in secret. Quinoa is called a grain but is actually the seed of a leafy plant. To me it is a grain in spirit. It is said to be a direct gift from the gods and if consumed daily could be a means of increased enlightenment. Although quinoa is relatively more expensive than other grains, it increases about three times its mass during the cooking process. It truly makes a little go along way, offers more iron than other grains, and contains high levels of potassium.

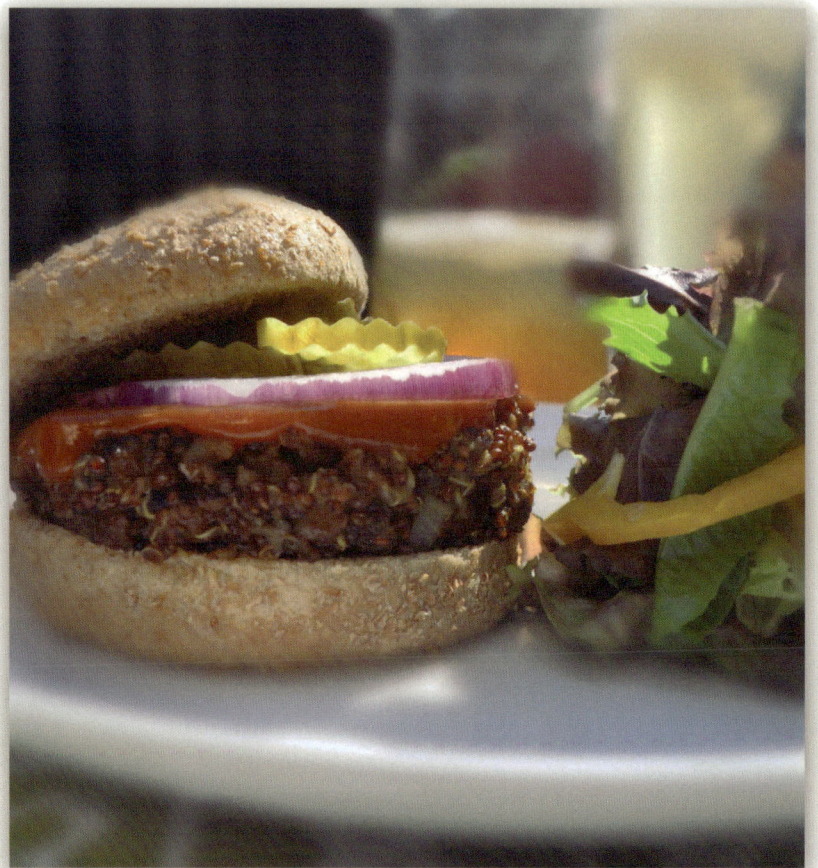

1 large eggplant
2 shallots, chopped fine
3 cloves garlic cloves, minced
1 teaspoon curry powder
½ teaspoon ground cumin
¼ teaspoon ground coriander
½ teaspoon smoked paprika
2 teaspoons arrowroot
1 teaspoon sea salt
½ teaspoon brown rice syrup
whole wheat buns, toasted
1 ½ cups water
1 bay leaf
¾ cup organic red quinoa, rinsed
1 cup red lentils, pre-soaked

Preheat oven to 425 °F.

Remove the top of the eggplant, and cut it in half lengthwise. Place cut sides down on a baking sheet lined with parchment paper. Bake for 25 - 30 minutes, or until the eggplant is tender.

Remove to a shallow dish, and allow to cool completely. While eggplant is cooking, in a medium saucepan, add 1 ½ cup water, bay leaf, and red lentils. Bring to a boil, and simmer for about 25 minutes, or until tender.

Soak the quinoa for 15 minutes in a medium saucepan. This will help to cook evenly, and loosens up the outer coating, which can give a bitter taste. Stir the quinoa with your hand, and pour off the rinsing water, using a fine mesh strainer.

In the medium saucepan, add 1 ½ cups cold water to the quinoa. Bring to a boil and cover with a tight fitting lid, turn heat down to a simmer for about 15 minutes. Remove from heat and let stand for 5 minutes. Fluff gently with a fork.

Once the eggplant is cool, discard any liquid that has accumulated, and scrape the flesh from the peel. Place the pulp in a food processor. Pulse a few times to make a coarse puree. Transfer to a medium-sized bowl; add the shallots, garlic, quinoa, lentils, curry, cumin, coriander, paprika, arrowroot, salt, and syrup. Mix well.

In a mixing bowl, add the Sloppy Sauce ingredients together and fold into the eggplant, lentil, quinoa mixture. Serve over top of toasted hamburger buns and add your favorite fixings.

SLOPPY SAUCE

2 cups ketchup
2 tablespoons mustard
1 tablespoon turbinado sugar
1 ½ tablespoons organic apple cider vinegar
1 tablespoon lemon juice, fresh squeezed
1 tablespoon shoyu

Musing No. 48

Making your dinners swoon-worthy only requires an open mind, a creative imagination, and a bit of whimsical notions.

SUNDAY PORTOBELLO BURGERS

serves 4

Keep an open mind when using mushrooms. Sometimes I do not know how a new recipe will evolve until I'm in the middle of it. Many times, I surprise myself with a delicious "accident," that unintentional dish that turned out better than anything I could have imagined. When working with Mother Nature's finest fungi (my daughter calls them "fairy homes"), your next "mistake" might just astound you.

4 large Portobello mushrooms, stems removed and gills scraped
½ cup red table wine
2 cloves garlic, chopped
3 shallots
sea salt and fresh ground pepper to taste (optional)
3 sprigs fresh thyme
8 whole wheat buns, toasted
½ large onion (optional)
1 bell pepper (optional)

Gently poke holes all over mushrooms. Place in a large baking dish.

Combine wine, garlic, shallots, and thyme and sea salt and pepper to taste in a saucepan and bring to a low boil. Allow to simmer for about 5 minutes. Pour this mixture on top of the mushrooms, coating each cap well. Cover and allow to marinate for about 2 hours.

Preheat broiler or pre-oiled grill. Remove mushrooms from marinade and discard liquid. Grill mushrooms on each side. Slather up the onion and bell peppers with a little olive oil, or any other favored veggie, and grill them along side your mushrooms.

Serve with your favorite burger fixings on toasted buns. This would be great paired with any green leafy salad or Herbed French Fries.

Musing No. 49

Mushrooms are one of those few plant sources that will provide you with vitamin D. They also offer plenty of potassium, selenium, and B vitamins.

KING NEPTUNE'S TRI-COLORED STUFFED PEPPERS
serves 6

This is one of those ways you can tuck in some of those must-have sea veggies. I got this recipe from my Aunt Jackie Drake-Clepper. She uses anchovies in her stuffed peppers, so the immediate thought to use seaweed in its place seemed like perfection, and perfection it is!

2 sheets of nori
6 cups veggie stock
2 cups brown rice
6 medium peppers, tri-colored
6 cups water or enough to just cover peppers
4 - 5 tablespoons olive oil
1 medium onion, finely chopped
2 cloves garlic, finely chopped
2 medium tomatoes, small dice
4 tablespoons white wine
⅓ cup parsley, chopped
sea salt and fresh ground pepper to taste

Preheat oven to 375 °F.

Toast nori on a dry baking sheet for 7 - 10 minutes or until crispy. Let cool and crumble; set aside.

In a large pot, over high heat, bring veggie stock to a boil. Add rice and stir. Turn heat to medium. Boil uncovered for about 25 - 30 minutes. Pour rice into a strainer and let set for about 20 seconds. Return rice to pot and cover with a tight-fitting lid. Allow to steam for about 10 minutes or until rice has absorb stock.

Uncover and fluff with fork. Season with salt. Pour rice onto a serving platter

Cut tops off the peppers. Scoop out the seeds. In a large pan of boiling water, blanch the peppers and their tops for about 5 minutes. Remove and cool upside down on a rack to drain.

In a large skillet pan, heat, oil, and sauté the onion and garlic until soft. Add in tomatoes and wine. Cook for about 5 minutes. Remove tomato mixture from heat. Stir in the rice and parsley. Stuff the peppers.

Top each pepper off with pre-toasted nori. Dust with freshly ground pepper and sea salt to taste.

BANG-BANG CHILI
serves 12

This Bang-Bang Chili is always, always a favorite in our home! It must be a southern thing. I made this for my daughter's 11th birthday party. She's my little Sagittarius (December baby) so it was chilly out. We had a bonfire, live music, friends, family, a henna artist, and, of course, a swami to read fortunes! Know what the most commented item on the party menu was? The Bang-Bang Chili. It was a hit with nothing left in the pot!

1 cup dried red kidney beans
4 cups water
1 cup bulgur
1 6-oz can tomato paste
2 bay leaves
6 cups vegetable broth
4 tablespoons olive oil
1 medium red onion, peeled, quartered and diced
1 red pepper, diced
1 green pepper, diced
1 jalapeno pepper, minced
2 - 4 thin slices fresh ginger, peeled
2 - 4 cloves garlic, peeled and minced
2 ½ teaspoons chipotle chili powder
2 teaspoons each: paprika, ground cumin, coriander
1 teaspoon each: dried thyme, basil, oregano
½ cup minced parsley or cilantro
2 ½ tablespoons Bragg's Liquid Aminos
3 - 4 teaspoons sea salt

KIDNEY BEANS
Soak dried, red kidney beans for 4 hours in hot water or overnight. This will help release some of the gases. Drain, rinse, and add 4 cups water. Bring to a boil, skim foam, cover, and simmer 2 hours.

CHILI
Add bulgur, tomato paste, bay leaves, and vegetable broth to kidney beans. Return to boil. Cover and simmer.

Sauté in pan over medium-high heat the oil, onion, red and green peppers, and jalapeno pepper for about 5 minutes. Add ginger, garlic, chili powder, paprika, ground cumin, coriander, and sauté 5 more minutes. Add thyme, basil, and oregano and sauté another 5 minutes.

Transfer the veggies to the bean and bulgur mix. Cook another 30 minutes.
Add parsley or cilantro and Bragg's Liquid Aminos. Add salt and pepper to taste. Also, add splashes of Bragg's to taste, if desired. Cook for a few more minutes and serve.

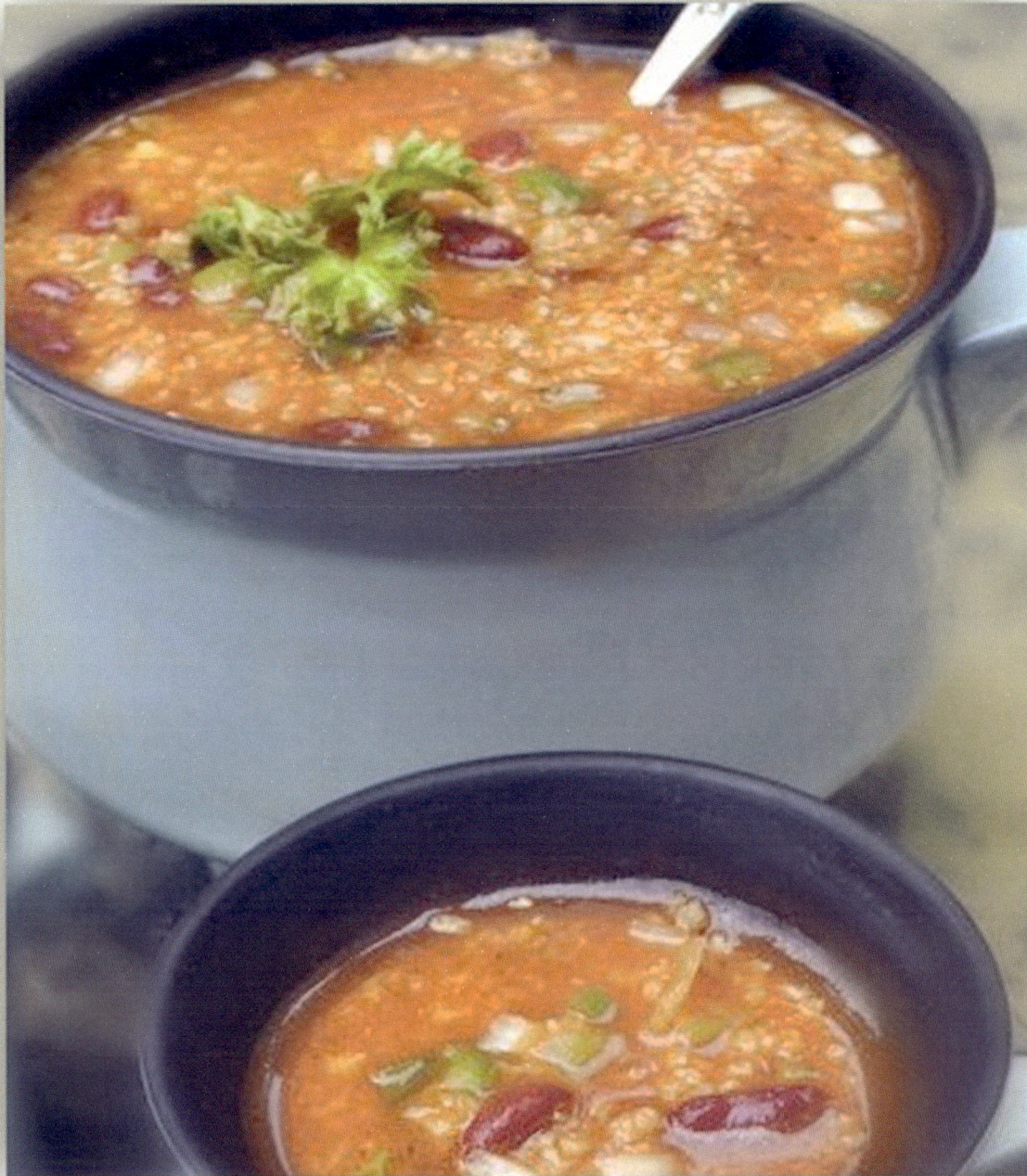

Musing No. 50

Dine a little greener everyday. If you are not vegan, try something new for yourself & incorporate some plant-based dishes into your meals or snacks.

POWER PASTA
serves 6

This is a powerful, cold pasta full of moxie and packed full of calcium, iron, and protein. I find that the boldness of this dish fits rather perfectly with the reason for this recipe in the first place: the power packed nutrients! This is one of those dishes that is lovely served in the warmer months, perhaps outdoors in your garden.

1 pound whole wheat pasta
2 ½ tablespoons olive oil
1 pound shelled frozen edamame
1 cup soybeans, pre-cooked
2 medium carrots, shaved
1 ½ tablespoons light miso paste
3 tablespoons hot water
4 scallions, chopped
1 teaspoon garlic, minced
¼ cup brown rice vinegar
3 tablespoons extra-virgin olive oil
Toasted nori with Sesame Seeds

Bring a large pot of salted water to a boil over high heat. Add pasta and cook, stirring occasionally until al dente, about 8 - 10 minutes. Drain and rinse under cold water to stop the cooking process. Toss with olive oil and set aside to cool.

In a pot of boiling water, add edamame and soybeans. Cook for about 4 - 5 minutes; drain and run under cold water.

With a vegetable peeler, make a pile of carrot shavings.

In a small bowl add miso paste and hot water. Mash miso paste until it has a liquid consistency.

In a large serving bowl, add the pasta, edamame, soybeans, carrots, scallions, garlic, liquid miso, vinegar and olive oil. Toss well mixture well. Sprinkle Toasted Nori with Sesame Seeds on top.

TOASTED NORI WITH SESAME SEEDS

2 - 3 sheets of nori
½ cup white sesame seeds

1 ½ teaspoons sea salt
1 teaspoon cayenne pepper

Toast the nori sheets by waving each sheet over a hot burner, and repeat until it becomes crisp. Use kitchen scissors to slice them into thin strips and then into squares. In a dry skillet over medium heat, toast sesame seeds slightly. With a mortar and pestle, grind seeds with sea salt until the seeds begin to adhere with the salt. Combine with cayenne pepper. Set aside.

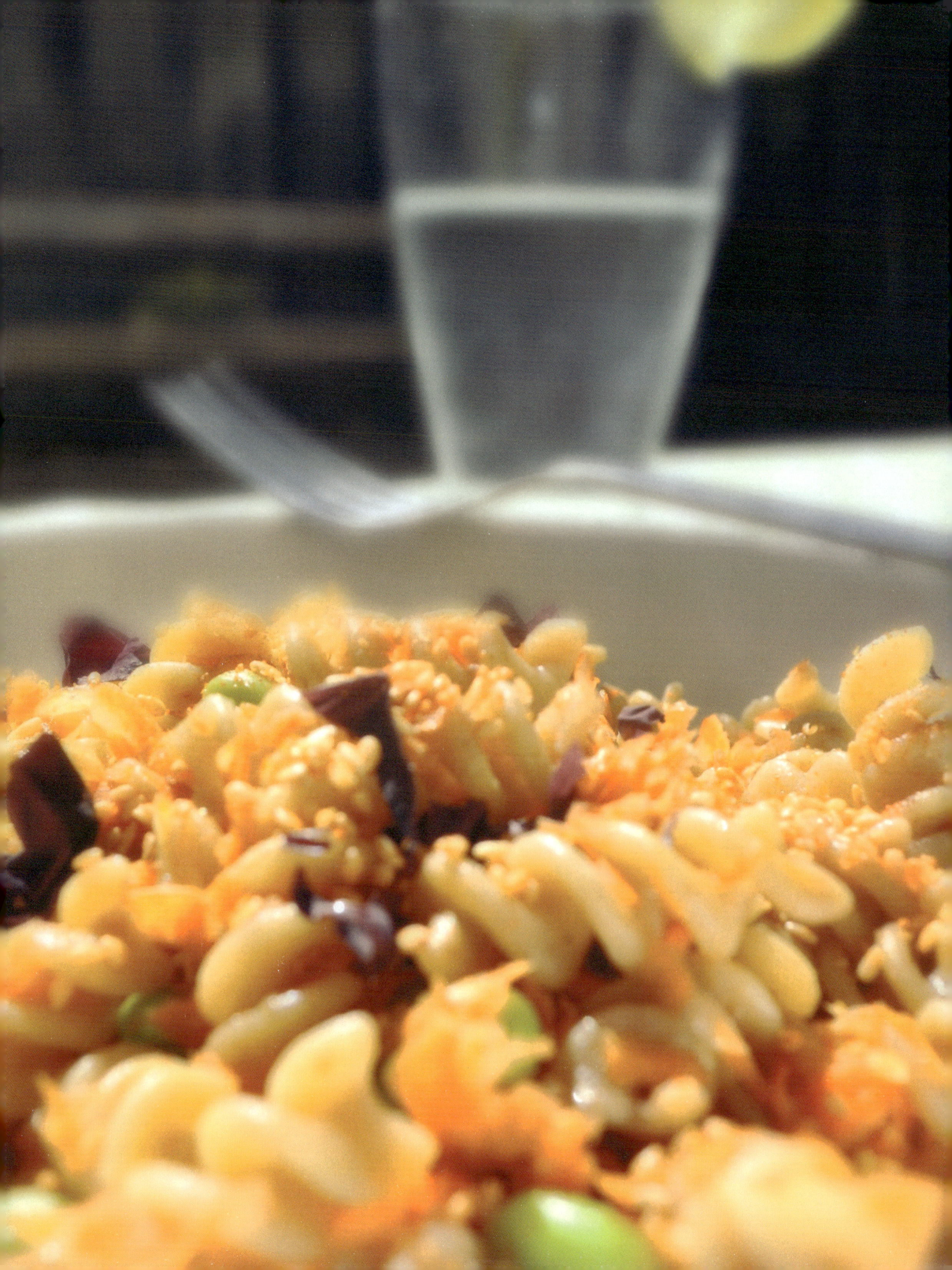

GRILLED RUSTIC PAELLA
serves 12

This is truly a must-have for your stash. To have a one-dish wonder to whip up and astound family and friends is priceless. Living a plant-based lifestyle does not mean you must give up on classic comfort foods. This is the result of many tried-and-tested vegan paellas.

1 teaspoon saffron threads
6 tablespoons extra virgin olive oil
1 large onion, diced
3 red bell peppers, cored, seeded and cut into strips
2 zucchini, cut diagonal into ¼ -inch thick slices
3 cloves garlic, minced
1 large handful parsley, rough chopped
1 tomato, cut into ¼ inch dice
1 ½ cups Arborio rice
1 cup garbanzo beans, pre-cooked
½ cup white wine
3 tablespoons paprika
¼ teaspoon cayenne
4 - 5 cups vegetable broth
sea salt and fresh ground pepper to taste
½ cup green peas

Place the saffron in a small bowl with 3 teaspoons of warm water and soak for a minimum of two hours. It can soak for as long as twelve hours, but two hours will give you the desired results.

When grill is ready, place your paella pan over the hottest area of the grill. Add olive oil to pan, sprinkle in the onion and heat until it sizzles. Add in the bell peppers and zucchini strips and cook over high heat, stirring until the onion begins to brown; this will take about 4 minutes. Add the garlic, parsley, and tomato.

Stir in the Arborio rice and cook until the grains look shiny, usually about 2 - 3 minutes. Add the garbanzo beans and cook for 1 - 2 minutes. Stir in drained saffron and white wine; let boil for about 1 minute. Stir in paprika, cayenne, vegetable stock, and season with salt and pepper to taste.

Move your paella pan farther away from the hot area to obtain a simmer. While simmering, add green peas and lightly toss paella pan to mix. Let the rice gently simmer until soft; this will take about 25 minutes. Add in the remaining broth, if needed. Do not stir the paella.

BAKED EGGPLANT CROWNED
WITH WHITE BEAN MASH

serves 4

1 large eggplant
2 ½ cups walnuts
1 cup bread crumbs
½ tablespoon dried oregano
1 tablespoon dried basil
2 garlic cloves, minced
sea salt and fresh ground pepper to taste
extra virgin olive oil for brushing
2 tomatoes, thinly sliced

Preheat oven to 350 °F. Line a baking sheet with Silpat or wipe down well with olive oil.

Slice eggplant into 4 ½-inch thick slices. Leave the peeling on and you will have a good amount of coating on the flesh of the eggplant.

Grind walnuts in food processor until powdered.

In a small bowl, mix bread crumbs, walnut powder, oregano, basil, garlic, and a pinch of salt and pepper. Brush both sides of the eggplant slices generously with olive oil. Dust eggplant with coating.

Place on the baking sheet; top each off with sliced tomato. Sprinkle with a bit more salt and pepper. Bake for 25 - 30 minutes.

Top with White Bean Mash and sprinkle any leftover fresh parsley.

WHITE BEAN MASH

1 - 2 large garlic cloves
¼ cup parsley
½ lemon grated
½ cup white beans, pre-cooked
extra virgin olive oil

Place all ingredients into a food processor, and drizzle in a little bit of olive oil.
Blend until creamy. Place a generous amount to the top of baked eggplant.

FRIDAY NIGHT PIZZA

serves 6 - 8

This is a weekend ritual, a must-do part of the weekend for us. We love the artistic release of creating a one-of-a-kind pizza. Dimming the lights, lighting candles, curling up in our cozy pj's, and popping in movies, just feels like a right of passage. Coming together for a calm eve of warm food, blissful banter, and familiar company completely changes ones state of mind and allows you to unwind into a weekend full of resting and relaxing for the week ahead.

DOUGH

4 ½ cups white whole wheat flour or whole wheat flour
1 ¾ teaspoons salt
1 teaspoon instant yeast
¼ cup extra virgin olive oil
1 ¾ cups ice water

Stir together the flour, salt, and instant yeast in the bowl of an electric mixer. By hand, stir in the oil and the cold water until it is all absorbed. Switch to the dough hook and mix on medium speed for 5 minutes, or as long as it takes to create smooth, sticky dough. The dough should clear the sides of the bowl but stick to the bottom of the bowl.

Add a in a little bit of water or flour to reach the proper consistency. You will want your dough to be springy and sticky. Transfer the dough to a floured countertop. Cut the dough into 6 equal pieces and mold each into a ball. Rub each ball with olive oil. Cover and refrigerate overnight.

PIZZA

cornmeal, for dusting
1 ½ cup cannelloni beans, pre-cooked and mashed
6 - 7 sun-dried tomatoes
2 – 3 garlic cloves, minced
1 teaspoon dried basil
1 teaspoon dried rosemary
1 large head radicchio, thinly sliced in ribbons
½ onion, thinly sliced
¼ teaspoon, raw cane sugar
1 – 1 ½ tablespoon extra-virgin olive oil
sea salt and fresh ground pepper to taste

When you are ready to make pizza, remove the desired number of dough balls from the refrigerator at least 1 hour before making the pizza. Make sure to keep them covered, so they don't become dry. At the same time, place a baking stone on a rack in the lower third of the oven.

Preheat the oven to 450 degrees.

If you do not have a baking stone, you can use the back of a sheet pan. Generously dust the back of a sheet pan with cornmeal, and get ready to shape your pizza dough.

Uncover the dough balls, and sprinkle them with a bit of flour. Begin to create a disk; you should be able to pull each round out to 12-inches or so. If the dough is being fussy and keeps springing back, let it rest for about 15 minutes.

Place the pulled-out dough on the prepared sheet pan, and make sure the dough will move around easily on the cornmeal, as you do not want your dough to stick.

In food processor blend white beans, sun-dried tomatoes, garlic, basil, and rosemary. Drizzle in a smidge of olive oil, if needed. Add this as the base of pizza for your "marinara." Pile on radicchio and onions and slide onto the baking stone.

About half way through, remove and sprinkle with raw cane sugar, which will produce a sort of caramelized layer to the toppings.

Bake until the crust is crisp and nicely colored. Remove from the oven.

I always finish with a small drizzle of extra virgin olive oil and dust with salt and pepper.

Musing No. 51

One way to add extra layers to your dishes, especially at dinner time, is to use aromatics, a bundle of herbs a.k.a. a bouquet garni. For my bundles, I use parsley sprigs, a couple of bay leaves, a few thyme sprigs, and a few sprigs of rosemary. Simply toss this mix into a cheesecloth bag and add to soups, stews, and rice. This will enhance the element of the cooking water & evoke an herbal scent to each dish.

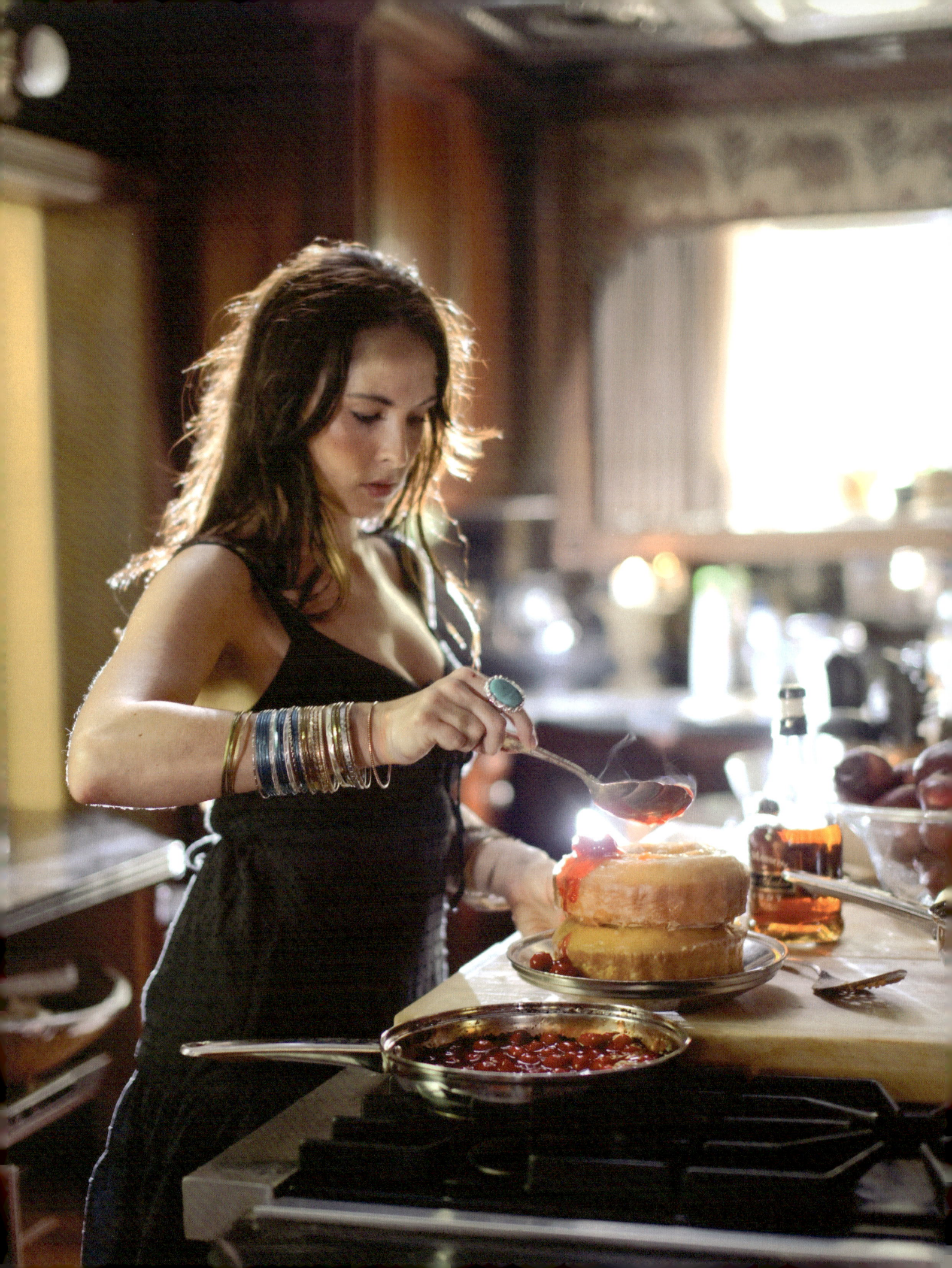

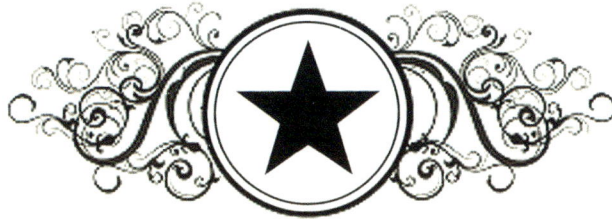

DESSERTS

One of my loves -- nay, obsessions -- is for all things rustically sweet. Then there is a craving for a decadent brownie with layers of chewy denseness drizzled with a light sweetness of brown rice syrup that is sure to make you love being a vegan. Fantasies and whims can be a great place to start when it comes to sweetened foods. Refine your tastes to a healthier, old world, simplicity. Create, imagine, and indulge.

POUND CAKE & CHERRIES FLAMBÉ

serves 6 - 8

I am ever-inspired by the many interesting events that unfold in this life we live. Never to take advantage & never to be ungrateful are two key components of my mindset. It warms my heart to create passionate & nostalgic moments that seem to kiss the memory forever. Lighting an after dinner desert on fire just seems to evoke my every whim and fantasy! Never take this very moment for granted, take it for what it is... a magical moment in time waiting for you to light up.

POUND CAKE

5 ounces organic silken tofu, drained well
⅔ cup raw cane sugar
¼ cup coconut oil
¼ cup vanilla soy milk
2 teaspoon pure vanilla extract
1 ½ cups white whole wheat flour
1 ½ teaspoon baking powder, aluminum free
1 teaspoon baking soda
½ teaspoon sea salt

Preheat oven to 350F. Wipe cake pan well with some coconut oil. Blend tofu, sugar, oil, milk, and vanilla extract in food processor until smooth.

Combine flour, baking powder, baking soda, and salt in large bowl. Fold in tofu mixture. Pour into cake pan, and bake 30 minutes or until toothpick inserted in center comes out clean.

Cool in pan 5 minutes, then un-mold and cool on wire rack until just warm.

GLAZE

⅓ cup confectioners sugar
1 tablespoon lime juice

Whisk together sugar and lime juice in small bowl until smooth. Drizzle over top of cake. Cool cake completely before serving to allow glaze to set.

CHERRY MIXTURE

1 10 ounce jar organic black currant jelly   ¼ cup brandy
2 cups Bing cherries, pitted

Place currant jelly in 9 inch skillet or shallow pan. Break up jelly with wooden spoon. Add cherries, reserve ¼ cup juice. Add drained cherries and ¼ cup juice to jelly. Stir using heat between medium and medium low. Heat uncovered until jelly has melted and sauce has come to rolling boil. Remove from heat.

Pour the cherry mixture over top of pound cake. In a small saucepan over medium heat, heat brandy. Carefully ignite the brandy, hold handle of lit brandy and pour overtop warm cherries and cake.

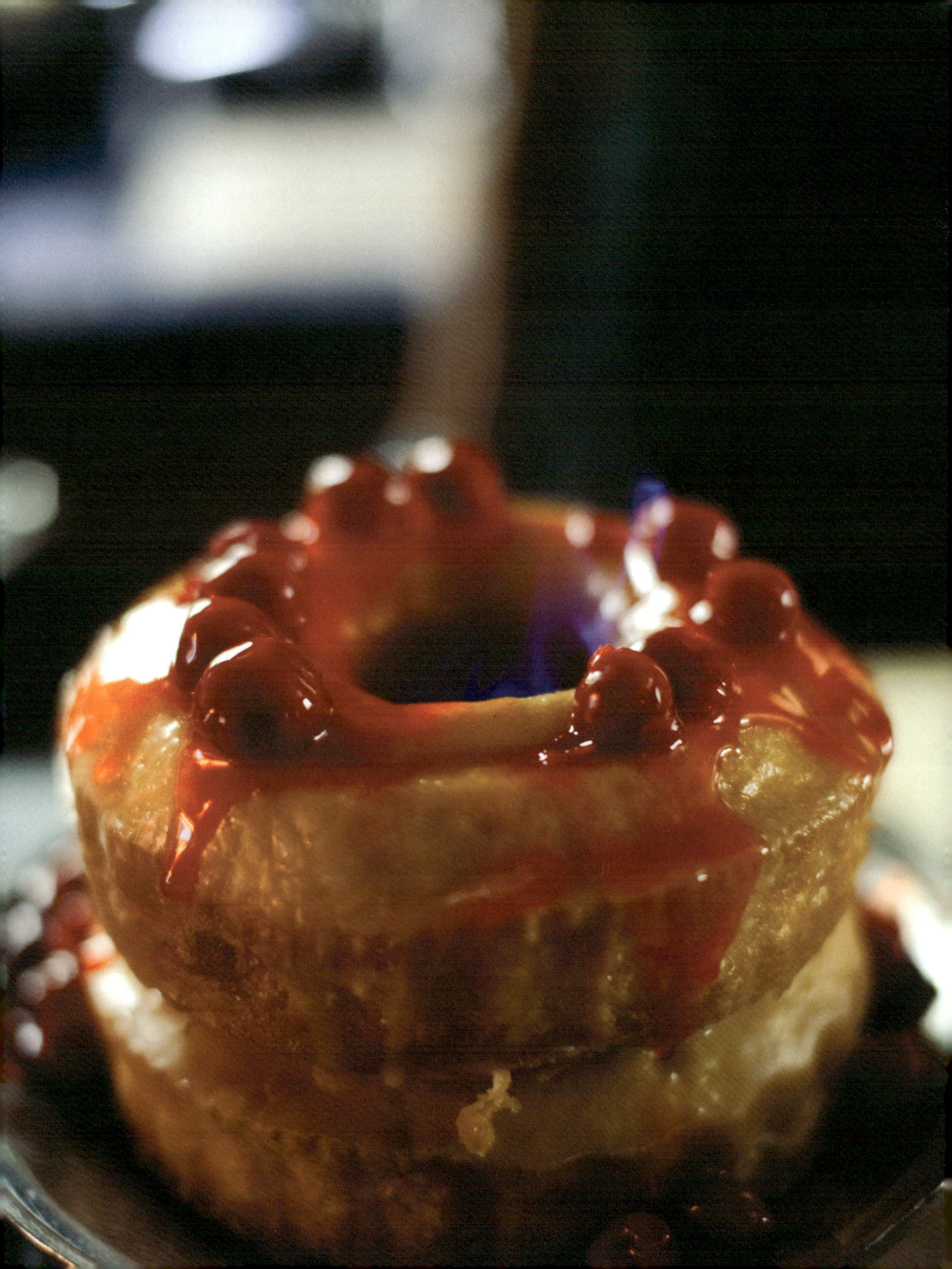

A BLONDIE MOMENT
serves 8

There is always room in ones repertoire for a quick-and-easy chewy dessert. These little blondies have got "the gams"! Note that these are not overly sweet but pack just the right amount of texture and flavor. Go on, have a blonde moment or two! If these are not sweet enough for you (I tend to gravitate more towards more earthy flavors) you can of course add a dollop of your favorite vegan ice cream and drizzle with brown rice syrup or vegan chocolate sauce.

1 can garbanzo beans, rinsed and drained
½ cup organic pineapple all-fruit spread
¼ cup tahini
2 teaspoons pure vanilla extract
¼ cup + 2 ¼ tablespoons flax meal
2 tablespoons oat flour
½ teaspoon baking powder, aluminum free
½ cup + ½ tablespoon raw cane sugar

Preheat the oven to 350 °F. Wipe down an 8-inch square baking pan lightly with coconut oil.

In a food processor, combine all ingredients, except for the ½ tablespoon of raw cane sugar. Blend until smooth. Pour mix into oiled pan, making sure the mixture is leveled.

Bake for about 25 minutes or until firm to the touch. Remove from oven.

Dust with ½ tablespoon raw cane sugar. Chill for a couple of hours before serving. Store in fridge.

Musing No. 52
Add a layer of fresh mint leaves to a dessert tray.

Musing No. 53
I am always inspired by the imperfections of life, by our many mistakes and by our many flaws. This is what pushes us into further understanding ourselves.

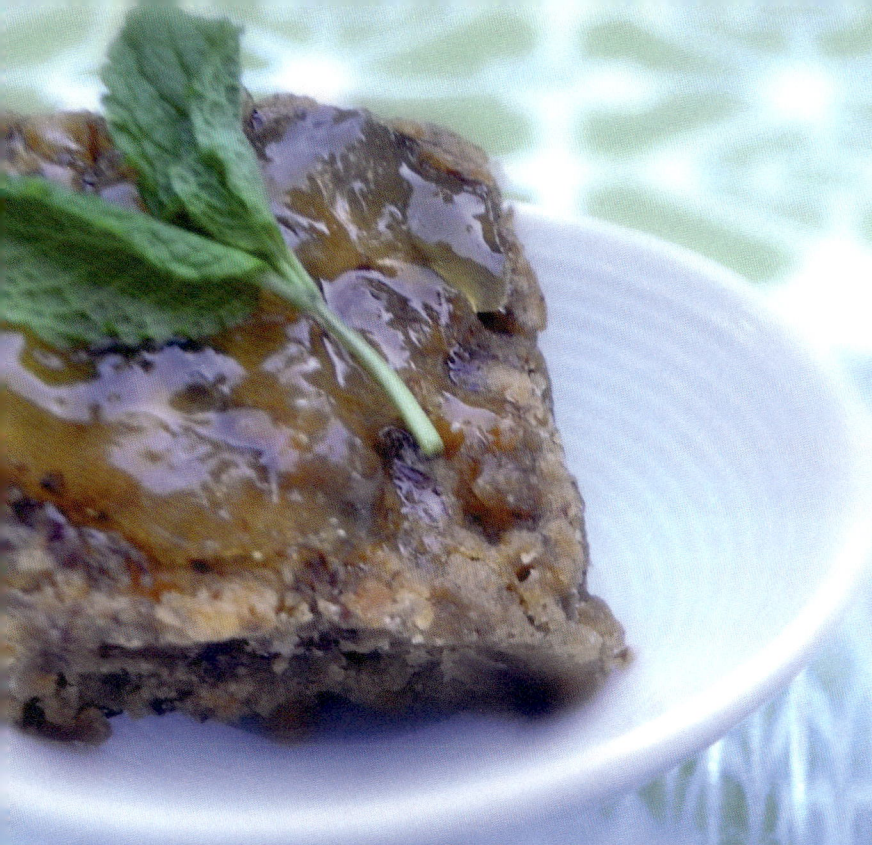

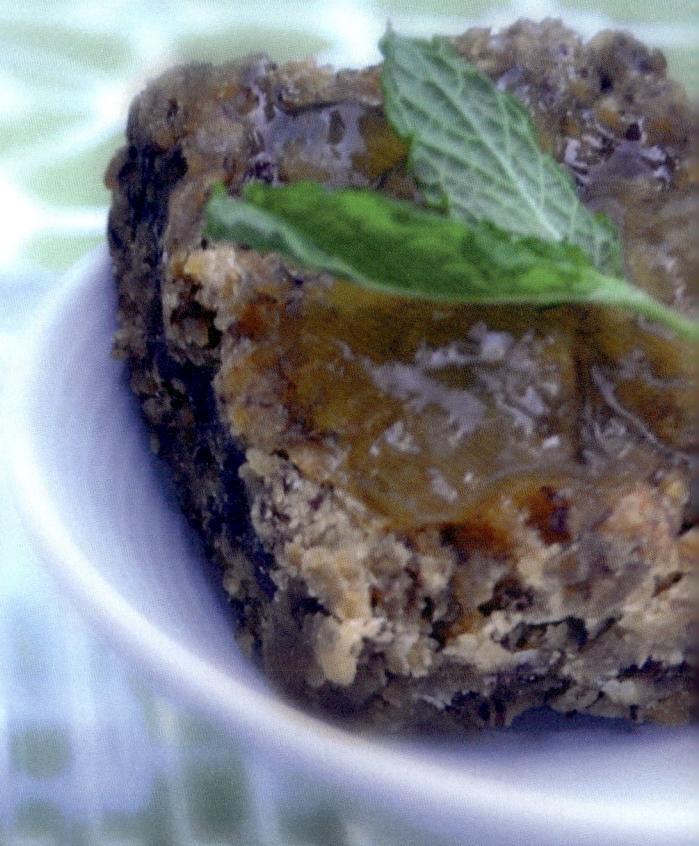

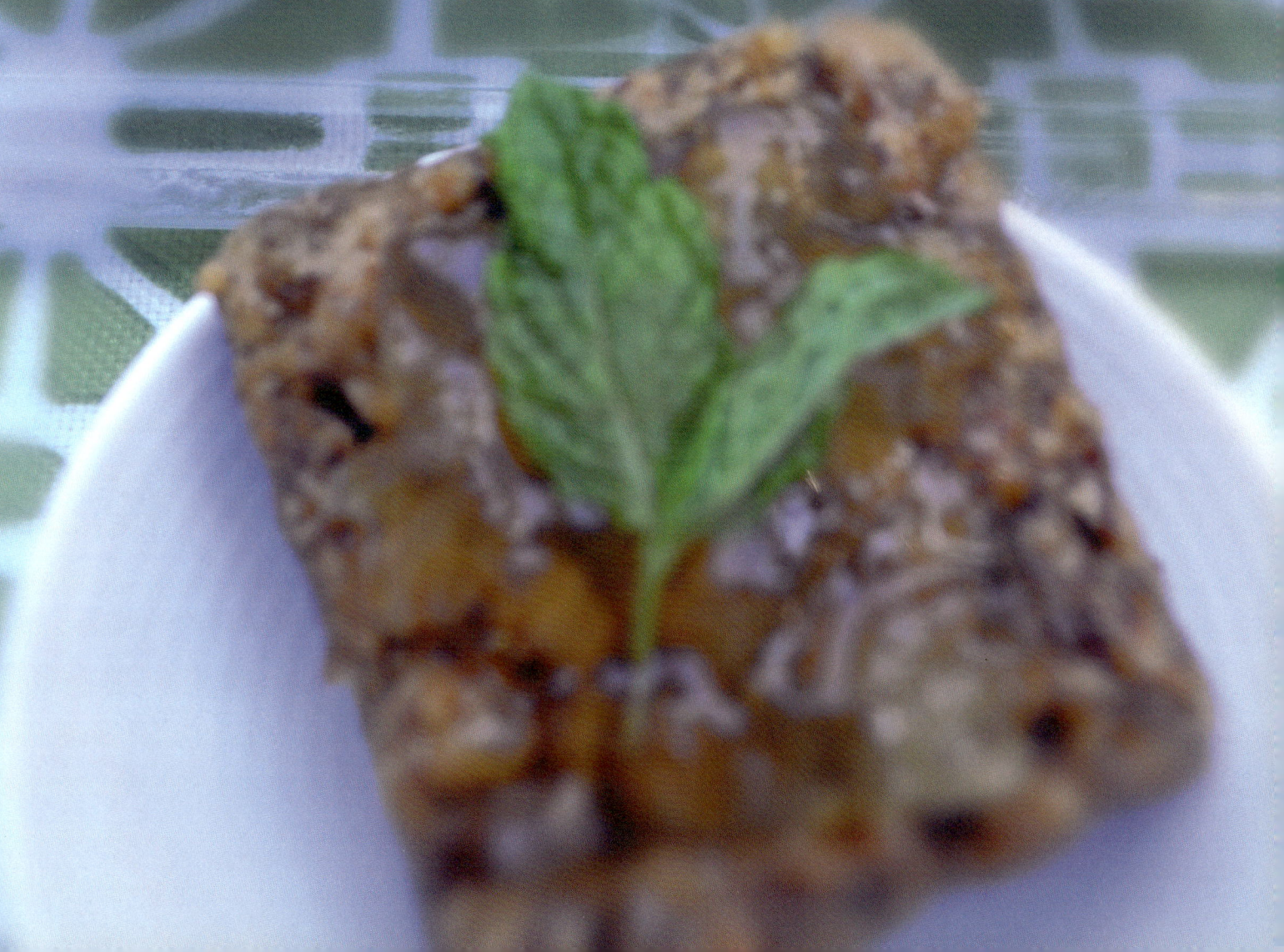

LAVENDER KISSED COOKIES

makes 20 cookies

Lavender comes from the Latin word lavare which means "to wash." This perfumed herb was used in bathing rituals by the Romans; the Egyptians used it for cooking and scenting the air. The offerings of this charmed herb are numerous. Discover its many diverse properties and indulge. These little cookies are an omen of many more batches to come. Simple, sweet, and earthy.

½ cup vegan butter
¾ cup raw cane sugar
3 teaspoons pure vanilla extract
1 ½ cups whole wheat pastry flour
½ teaspoon baking soda
½ baking powder, aluminum free
2 teaspoons arrowroot
¼ teaspoon fine sea salt
2 tablespoons culinary dried lavender
2 tablespoons coconut milk

Preheat oven to 350° F. Wipe 2 baking sheets with coconut oil.

In a large bowl mix together the vegan butter and sugar. Stir in vanilla. In a separate mixing bowl, sift together the flour, baking soda, baking powder, arrowroot, and salt. Fold in the lavender.

Stir the dry ingredients into the wet. Add the milk, as needed: you will not want your dough to be too wet or too dry.

Divide the dough into twenty equal sections using a heaping tablespoon of dough. Place on pre-oiled baking sheets. With fork, flatten dough down a little bit, as the cookies will not spread while baking. This will also give the cookies a nice little print.

Bake for 15 minutes or until the edges are golden brown.

If you want these kissed gems to be chewier, bake for only 10 minutes or so. Wait a minute or two before transferring them over to a serving platter.

Musing No. 54

Let the charms of divine, compassionately created sweets take hold.

GENIE GEMS

makes 12-14 cookies

A light, chewy gem that I swear promotes a small level of cosmic consciousness. According to legend, offering sesame to Lord Ganesha was a must and considered the most auspicious oil next to Ghee. The phrase "open sesame" was inspired by the glory of the sesame seed's pod, which bursts open when it reaches its ultimate maturity stage. Serve with a diffusion of herbal tea, sweetened with agave, and creamed with almond milk. This combination of perfect synergy is sure to offer up its sweet charms.

1 cup whole wheat pastry flour
1 cup cooking oats,
the quick cooking kind
1 cup turbinado sugar
½ teaspoon baking soda
¼ teaspoon Himalayan sea salt
¼ cup black sesame seeds
½ cup golden raisins
¼ cup tahini
2 tablespoons sesame oil
½ cup almond or hemp milk
1 teaspoon pure vanilla extract
¼ cup fruit preserves or
chutney, for topping
2 tablespoons brown rice syrup,
for drizzling

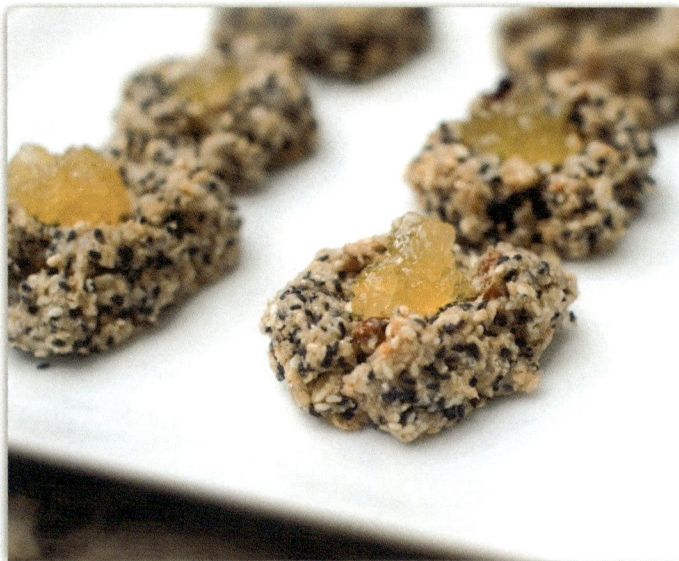

Preheat oven to 375°. Wipe down 2 baking sheets with oil.

In a medium bowl, whisk together flour, oats, sugar, baking soda, salt, sesame seeds, and golden raisins.

In a small bowl, whisk together the tahini, oil, milk, and vanilla. Stir the wet ingredients into the dry. If the dough is too dry, just add a bit more milk.

Divide the dough into 12 equal portions, about 2 tablespoons of dough.

Place on the pre-oiled baking sheet. With a spoon, press down into each cookie, as these will only spread a little during baking and this will add a nice little nook for a dollop of your favorite fruit preserves or chutney.

Bake for about 10 minutes or until set. Wait about 10 minutes before transferring them to a rack to cool. Spoon on your favorite fruit spread and drizzle lightly with brown rice syrup.

PEACE PIE
serves 8

A recipe for achieving a peace mind is worth more than all of the gems in the world. Yoga poses that evoke a feeling of bliss mixed with intense concentrations of focusing on ones awareness with meditation and surrounding yourself with nature are the basic mix of ingredients to find inner peace. Inner peace is the connection of your whole mind and body. It will enhance one's life experience, thus creating a calming comfort that is sure to inspire others. Be a muse, create your own recipe for inner peace, and discover the divine flow of life.

1 ¼ cups light spelt flour
2 ounces unsweetened nondairy bittersweet chocolate, finely chopped
¼ cup raw cane sugar
¼ teaspoon baking powder, aluminum free
¼ teaspoon fine sea salt
½ teaspoon cinnamon
¼ cup almond oil
3 tablespoons hemp milk

Preheat oven to 375 degrees. In a food processor, blend the flour, chocolate, sugar, baking powder, salt, and cinnamon. Add the oil, about 1 tablespoon at a time, and pulse with each spoonful. Add the milk, 1 tablespoon or so at a time, until dough begins to form.

Shape the dough into a ball. Chill for 2 hours. After dough has chilled, roll out (sprinkle work surface with flour) to about a 12 inch round.

Transfer dough to a pre-oiled baking pan. If your dough tears, just pinch it back into place. Crimp and style your dough around pan. Set aside and make the filling.

FILLING

2 cups cashews, ground
⅔ cup mirin
¼ teaspoon sea salt
¼ cup hemp milk
2 ½ tablespoons dark rum
1 teaspoon pure vanilla extract
1 teaspoon ground cinnamon
1 teaspoon ground nutmeg

In a mixing bowl, combine the ground cashews, mirin, and salt. Stir the milk, rum, vanilla, cinnamon, and nutmeg until combined. Pour filling into the crust and level out with a spoon. Bake for about 25 minutes.

Drizzle with your favorite chocolate syrup and dust with finely chopped cashews. This pie is best served chilled.

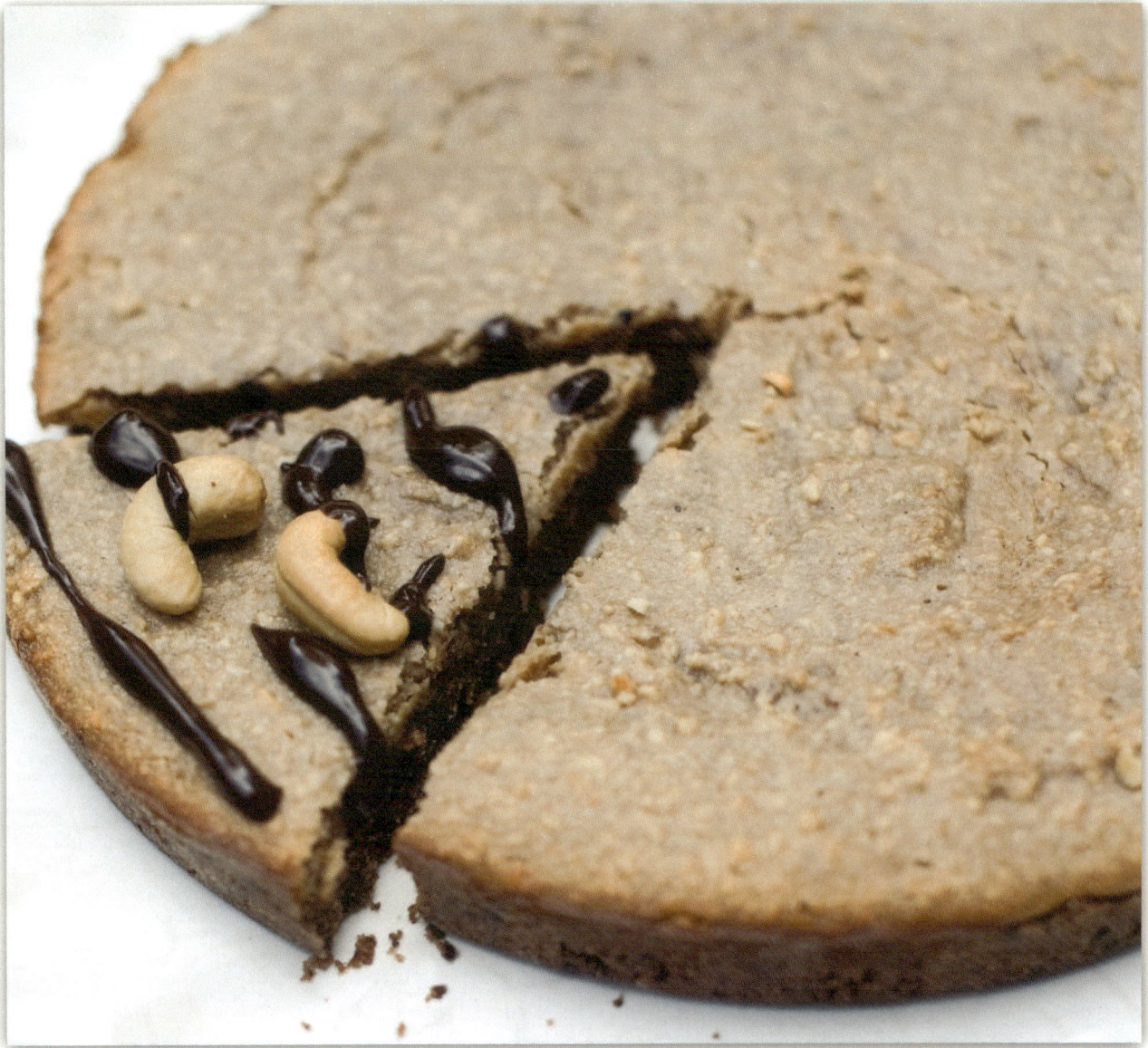

Musing No. 55

Freeze mint sprigs in ice-cube trays & serve in decorative bowls to refresh water or cocktails.

TUATHA DE DANANN BROWNIES

serves 6-8

This is the stuff dreams are made of... well, mine anyways! I had always made my brownies with my standby recipe and then drizzled brown rice syrup overtop for an added wickedly divine sweetness. But for this book, I wanted to re-think my original. Although the original was demure and wonderful, I wanted her a bit more decadent and obscure! By simply adding the brown rice syrup into the batter, it's like waving a magic wand over them. Cheers to your magic kitchen wand moments!

¾ cup whole wheat flour
¼ teaspoon baking soda
¼ cup cocoa powder
⅛ teaspoon salt
½ (12 ounce) package organic tofu, drained
¼ cup coconut oil
1 cup turbinado sugar
4 teaspoons vanilla extract
4 (1-ounce) squares bittersweet chocolate, chopped
½ cup + 2 tablespoons almond milk
½ cup dark chocolate chips
¼ cup brown rice syrup

Preheat oven to 350 °F.

Oil an 8-inch square pan. Combine flour, baking soda, cocoa powder, and salt in a bowl; stir well. Place the tofu into a blender. Cover, and puree until smooth. Add the oil and sugar. Blend for about 30 seconds; pour into a mixing bowl and stir in the vanilla extract.

Melt the bittersweet chocolate in the top of a double boiler over just-barely simmering water, stirring frequently. Add in the 2 tablespoons of almond milk. Scrape down the sides with a rubber spatula to avoid scorching.

Mix the melted chocolate into the tofu mixture until well blended. Stir in flour mixture until thoroughly combined, about 1 minute. Add in about ½ cup almond milk. Fold in the chocolate chips and brown rice syrup; blend well.

Pour mix into pre-oil pan and bake in the preheated oven until a toothpick inserted into the center comes out clean, about 30 minutes. Cool before slicing into bars.

For added sweetness, drizzle brown rice syrup over top of cooled brownies.

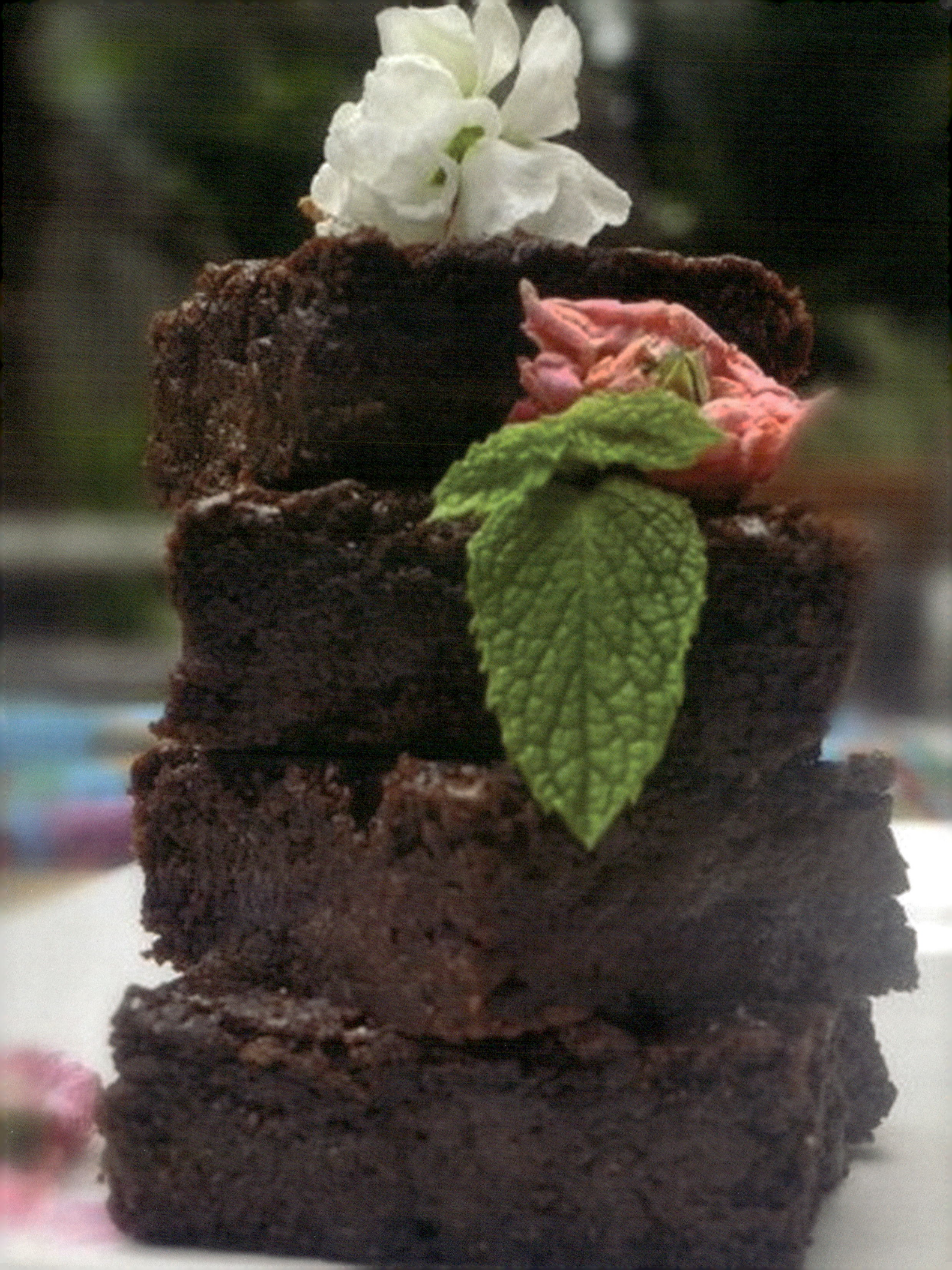

SWEET TAHINI YOGINI BARS
makes 6 bars

A yogini is the term for a female yoga practitioner. A yogini evokes an effect to create extraordinary change within themselves as well as the world around. The bliss of a yogini is to live a life dedicated to the knowledge of conscious insights, spiritual awareness, and producing a well sweetly balanced life full of divine experiences. I am quite smitten with the sweet balance of the tahini, spices, chocolate, and healthy goodness of the brown rice and barley in this quick little sweet.

¼ cup agave nectar
3 ¼ tablespoons tahini
2 ounces non dairy dark chocolate, chopped
1 ½ teaspoon pure vanilla extract
1 cup wheat and barley cereal
2 cups crispy brown rice cereal

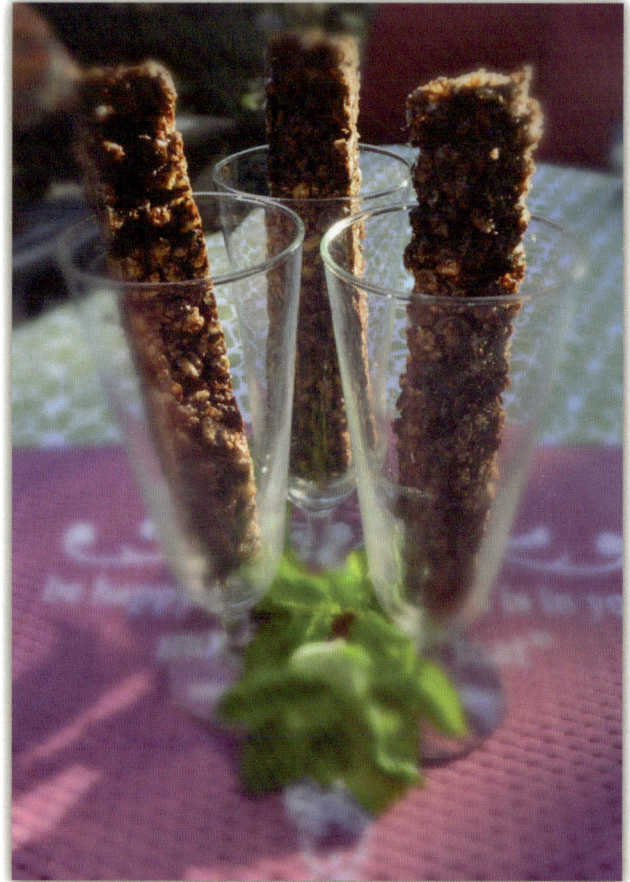

Wipe an 8-inch square baking dish with coconut oil.

Combine agave, tahini, and chocolate, and melt over a low heat in a double broiler until completely melted, stirring consistently. Add the allspice, vanilla, and cereals; mix well.

Pour into the pre-oiled pan, making sure it is leveled.

Place in the freezer to set. Slice into bars, and serve.

Musing No. 56
Ever tried brown rice syrup? Drizzle over cakes & such. It is a wonder to behold!!

GLITTERING GRAPES SCENTED WITH ROSE WATER

serves 10

It is said that Old World alchemists were responsible for introducing rose water to the world. The creation of this seductive concoction is quite simple and can be made at home by a process of steam distillation. Since the dawn of time, many folks have relied on homemade remedies for ailments. Their gardens of herbs, vegetables, and apothecary roses gave them the ingredients needed. Rose water offers up the power to relieve depression by simply adding its essential oil to the bath. As a compress it can soothe headaches and has assisted in the healing of sunburns and wounds. This fragrant, magical water is quite divine to have around and can offer its wonder in the most unexpected recipes. Create these little ornaments for a festive gathering: glittery bouquets that will offer an unexpected perfumed kiss of the rose water.

3 - 4 large bunches of red grapes
1 - 2 cups rose water
1 cup raw cane sugar, vegan white sugar, or turbinado sugar

Place grape bunches into a large bowl and pour rose water over top. Adjust grapes so that all are submerged. Let stand for 25 - 30 minutes.

Pour sugar into a casserole dish. Remove grapes and roll into dish of sugar, coating well.

Place glittered grapes onto a platter and freeze for 30 minutes. Remove glittered baubles onto a serving platter.

Musing No. 57

Garnish cupcakes with edible sugared flowers for old world charm.

Musing No. 58

Want a perfumed kiss? Try soaking grapes in Rosewater.

Musing No. 59

Create some magic this eve & have dessert in bed!

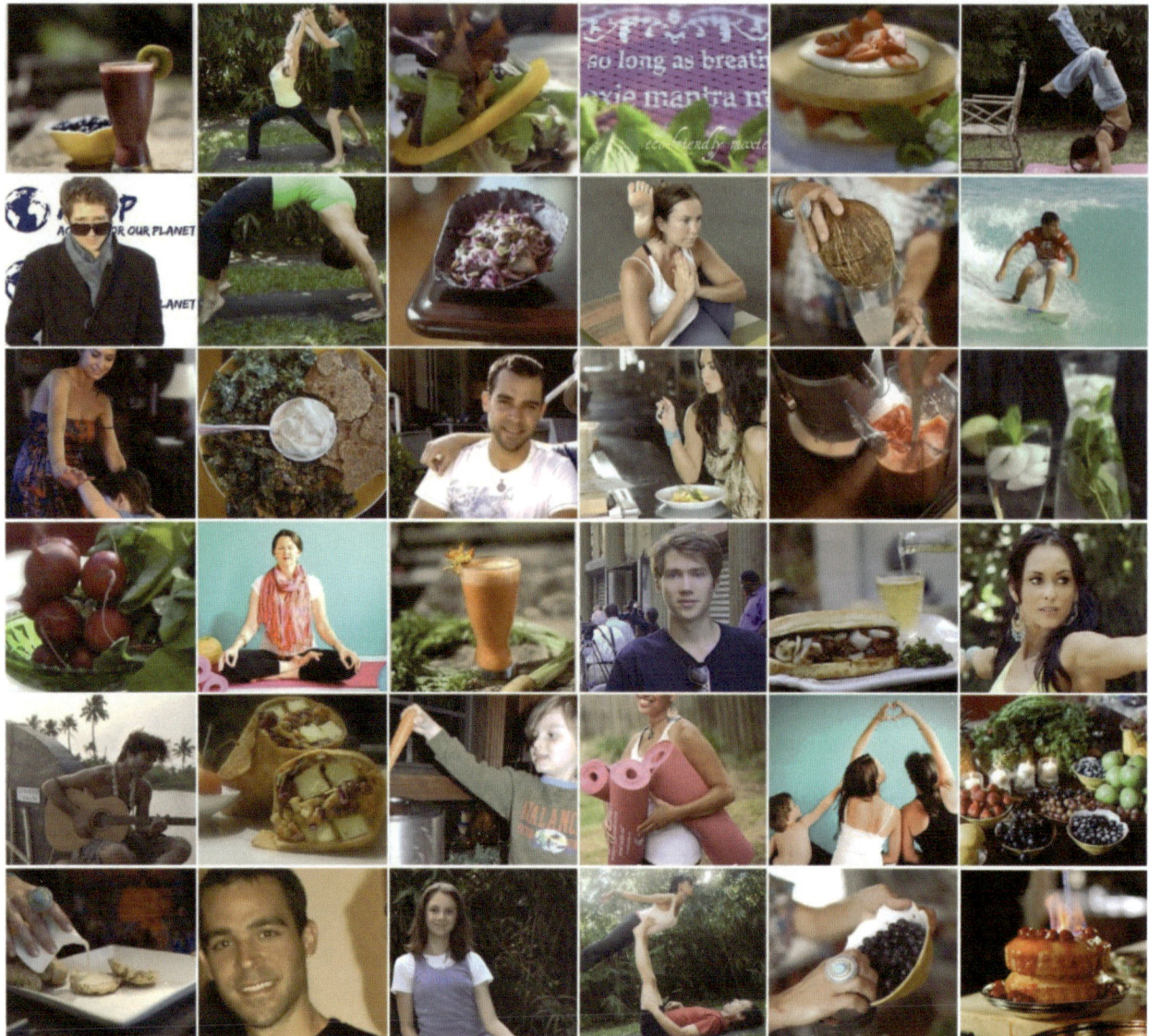

Offerings from the friends of the vegan muse

A collection of recipes & inspirations for you to enjoy & be uplifted by

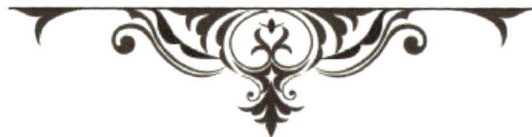

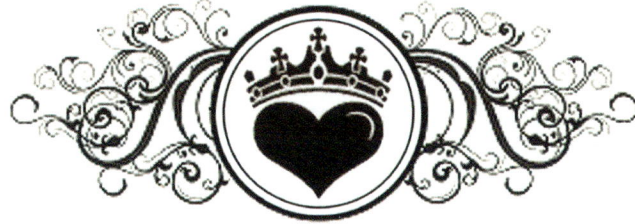

FEATURED FRIENDS

FEATURED FRIENDS, A.K.A. FORAGERS OF GOODNESS AND COMPASSION, JOINED HANDS FROM ACROSS THE GLOBE TO OFFER THEIR FAVORITE PLANT-BASED RECIPES, MUSINGS, THOUGHTS, AND YOGIC INSPIRATIONS.

Ann Kiyonaga-Razon, RYT 200 hour, hails from in St. Augustine, Florida (famous for being the oldest city in the US!) with her husband, Didier, and their two sons, Joseph and Paul. She holds a master's degree in international studies from the Johns Hopkins School of Advanced International Studies. Shortly after receiving this degree, she had a mystical experience through an encounter with a meditation master, which led to the great good fortune of spending eleven and a half years in an Indian ashram (monastery).

The mystical life lends itself to the language of poetry. Thus, naturally, Ann eventually found herself drawn to this beautiful art form. Aside from writing poetry, Ann has offered readings, taught poetry classes to both adults and children, and presented her "Touch the Poet Within" workshop. Additionally, she served as the Poetry Facilitator for monthly gatherings at the local Barnes and Noble over a two-year period.

Ann is also a yoga teacher, a profession she enjoys immensely as (aside from the obvious physical benefits) yoga naturally encourages and uplifts. She helps offer the Two Suns Rising Yoga Teacher Training, RYT 200 hour, with her husband, Didier Razon, RYT 500 hour. Her specialties are a series of guided contemplations and meditations which she calls Journey to the Heart, as well as finding ones voice as a yoga teacher. "I like to also discusses how to create a balanced yoga class as well as a personal lifestyle - like a good story - with a beginning, middle and end, as well as the use of themes to create and organize ones yoga class or ones life." You can find many inspirations from Ann via her website, www.graceofthehearthealing.com

The heart is the hub of all sacred places. Go there and roam.~ Bhagavan Nityananda

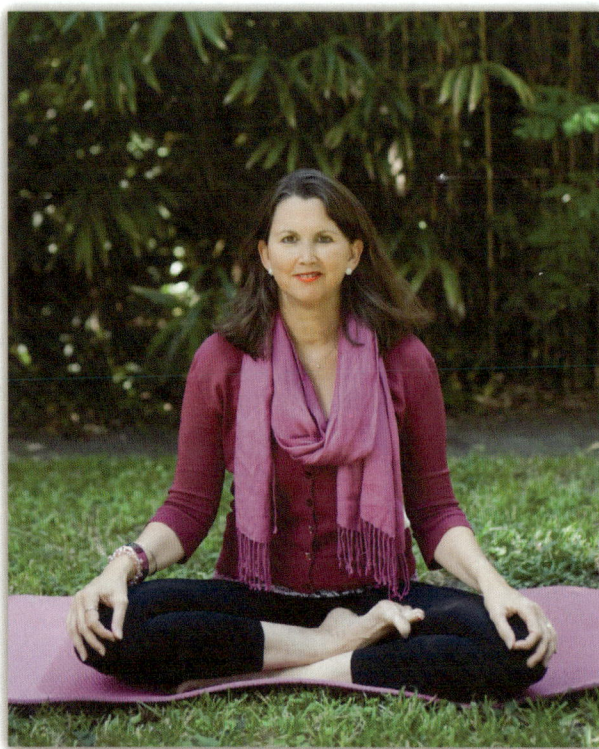

Musing No. 60

A yogini embraces her spiritual growth, her dreams & visions.
She is a world changer.

ROSE WATER

This recipe will make enough to have some to store for many uses.

One of Ann Kiyonaga-Razon's favorite fragrances to wear is rose water…simply elegant, beautifully fresh, and evokes a feminine touch. Dab on pulse points, sprinkle on lingerie, pour into a bath, the uses are endless. Makes for a nice, all natural, cruelty-free fragrance.

1 brick
stockpot
2 -4 quarts distilled water
10 cup rose petals
small heat-proof bowl, to sit on top of brick
heat-proof bowl, used to tightly cover stockpot
ice cubes

Place brick in the bottom of stock pot. Place rose petals around the exterior of brick.

Pour water over top until petals and brick are submerged and just covered. Place small heat-proof bowl securely on top of the brick. Bring the water and petals to a boil. Lower heat and simmer.

Place a heat-proof bowl tightly on stockpot, one that is large enough to tightly seal the pot. Fill the heat-proof bowl with ice cubes. Allow petal mixture to continue to simmer for about 3 ½ hours.

Replace ice as it melts. When done, the collecting bowl will hold the rosewater and will have a thin layer of rose oil. This oil may be separated from the water and used as essential oil.

Allow to cool. Funnel into a sterilized glass bottle or jar. Refrigerate and use within a few days.

Use as a spritz for body, or in bathwater.

Musing No. 61

There are no imperfections…just originality.

Musing No. 62

Sweet dreams tonight I shall keep
with fragrant herbs tucked beneath my sheet.

Kelly Green, RYT 500 hour, hails from Ft. Lauderdale, Florida, Kelly cultivates an amazing life with her husband, Chris, and two children, Ashley and Austin. Her home studio is the location of the well known Barkan Method. She began yoga in 2003 and has been teaching since 2004. She trained under Jimmy Barkan's Level I, II, and III hot yoga flow as well as many other styles of yoga.

She is influenced by Ashtanga, Anusara, Jivammukti, and, of course, her guru Jimmy Barkan but most of all by her students. As one of his top teachers, she assists him with his Level II Teacher Training bringing another dynamic to his teaching style and travels around the world teaching workshops and retreats. Born with birth defects in her knees later resulting in an injury brought her on this yogic path. Her goal is to share the healing power of yoga with as many people as possible. Kelly's passion for yoga shows in all that she does. "Yoga is not just a 60- 90 minute practice; it is a way of life.

The yoga practice is a life practice. The real postures begin once you step off your mat." She is forever grateful for the many gifts along the way that yoga has given and the many lessons it has taught. "I share an amazing life with my other half, Chris, and his two children, Ashley and Austin. I am so lucky to have so many people in my life that love me - family, friends, and students. I enjoy a challenging yet very compassionate yoga routine."

Learn how to truly "live" your yoga, not just "practice" it. Each posture, breath, and class should make you feel more inspired and stronger than the next.

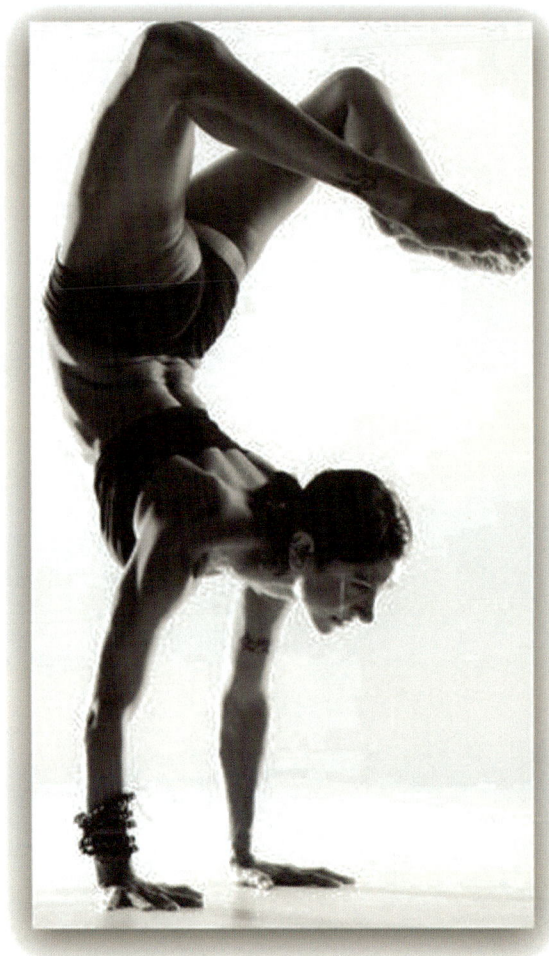

YOGINI POWER BARS

serves 4

This fabulous get-up-and-go bar doesn't take a lot of time to make. Layers of crunchy whole grains and natural sweet flavors can create a quick snacking alternative, rather than your standard prepackaged bars that have ingredients that cannot be pronounced. It's all about the balance of textures and flavors with this little quickie.

4 teaspoons flax meal
1 ½ tablespoons water (warm is best)
2 tablespoons agave nectar
½ teaspoon pure vanilla extract
2 tablespoons + 1 teaspoon brown rice flour
⅛ teaspoon baking powder, aluminum free
⅛ teaspoon baking soda
⅛ teaspoon sea salt
1 cup almonds, coarsely chopped
½ cup dried coconut shreds
½ cup dried cranberries

Preheat oven to 350 °F. Lightly coat an 8 x 4-inch loaf pan with coconut oil.

In a small bowl, whisk together the flax meal and water until combined. Add the agave and vanilla; stir well.

In a medium bowl, combine the flour, baking powder, baking soda, salt, almonds, coconut, and dried fruit. Fold the wet ingredients into the dry. Pour mixture into pan and press down firmly with back of spoon.

Bake for 25 minutes or until golden brown. Keep in pan and allow to cool. Remove from pan and cut into bars.

Musing No. 63

A yogini believes in herself and thus has power.

Musing No. 64

The New pretty is…confident, liberated, and soulful.

Tara Rawson, RYT 200 hour, and an ambassador for Lululemon, hails from Jacksonville, Florida and is a wife, mother, yogini, mystic, and inspirational teacher to many. She is the co-owner of Ananda Kula and Director of its yoga school, leading workshops, kirtans, and teacher training programs. Her Sadhana, or yogic practice, is steeped in Tantric philosophy, weaving love, light, and consciousness in all her endeavors on and off the mat.

 Tara has a daily practice of asana, pranayama, meditation, and mantra, which allows her to bring her experience and insight directly to her students with love and sincerity. What she loves most about her practice is the presence that comes through regular meditation, mantra, and devotional chanting. Her passion and life work is to be a vehicle that carries healing light and consciousness to transform the lives of those around her. More information on Tara's yogini lifestyle can be found at www.yogaanandastudio.com

When you are inspired by some great purpose, some extraordinary project, all your thoughts break their bounds. Your mind transcends limitations, your consciousness expands in every direction, and you find yourself in a new, great, and wonderful world.
~ Patanjali

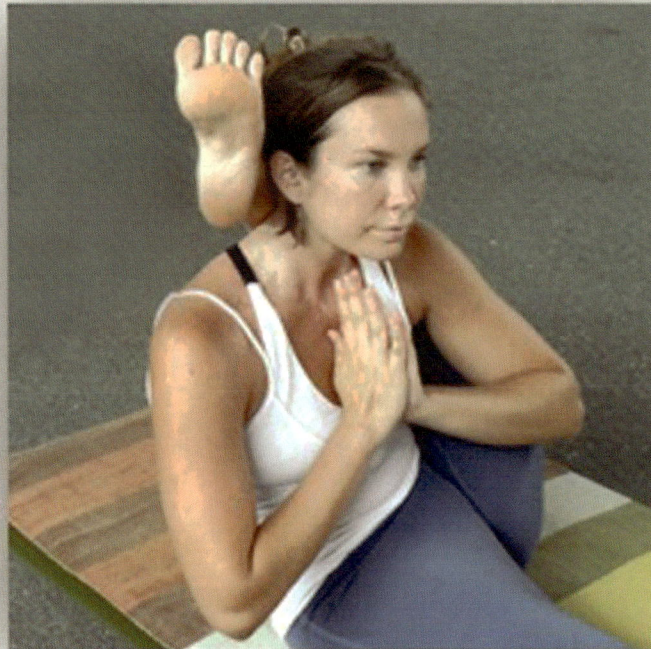

Musing No. 65

Her only fear is convention. Her only weakness is nature & selfless works…her life has a purpose, to grow, love, and learn.

BAREFOOT GIRLS INVIGORATING
TOOTSIE TONIC

Kick off your shoes, roam barefoot, and feel the earth underneath. Let the candle wax drip where it may. Enjoy your strengths, and feel the beauty from within. Rest your mind and body, soothe your soul, and lift your spirits.

4 - 5 drops lavender essential oil
2 drops tea tree essential oil
5 drops rosemary essential oil

Fill a basin or a large bowl with warm water. Add essential oils. Soak feet and enjoy. Take deep breaths in and out of the nose. Take this time for a mini-meditation vacation! Soak for 10 - 15 minutes. Add more warm water if desired

BEET STAINED BEAUTY

Want a cruelty-free and creative way to tint and moisturize those puckers? This is my all time favorite way to create a one of a kind lip balm. I have a little area in my bathroom that I can keep these entire ingredients ready available to make more on demand!

1 ½ tablespoons coca butter, warmed (I have also used coconut butter)
2 drops of oil of eucalyptus
1 ½ teaspoons beet powder (you can find this at Whole Foods Market or your local health market. If they do not have it, simply ask and they should be able to order some!)

Light a small candle.

Place your butter into a small bowl or saucer and hold up over the candle and heat. When warmed add drops of oil and beet powder and mix well. Pour into a small container and allow to cool.

Rub finger into your balm and apply generously.

Musing No. 66

Use mashed avocado for a moisturizer. Massage onto hands thoroughly and allow to sit for about 20 minutes before rinsing with warm water.

Kimberli Hargnett, RYT 200 hour, hails from Orange Park, Florida and is the founder and owner of Life's Journey Yoga & Wellness. She has years of experience in Holistic Wellness combined with a heart for helping others reach higher levels of health. After being trained in the Kripalu Yoga technique at Discovery Yoga in St. Augustine, FL, Kimberli opened Life's Journey's doors with a mission to offer the type of yoga instruction and awareness that would assist individuals through life's turbulent emotions and health issues.

The positive changes Kimberli began experiencing due to yoga and other forms of natural health fueled her passion to help people in her community also heal and reach their fullest potential: spiritually, emotionally, mentally, and physically. Today, with the assistance of a team of yoga instructors, a variety of yoga and wellness services are offered at Life's Journey Yoga & Wellness. Kimberli's Art Healing class is the most recent addition to the line-up of classes and workshops. More information on Kimberli's yogini lifestyle can be found at www.lifesjourneywellness.com

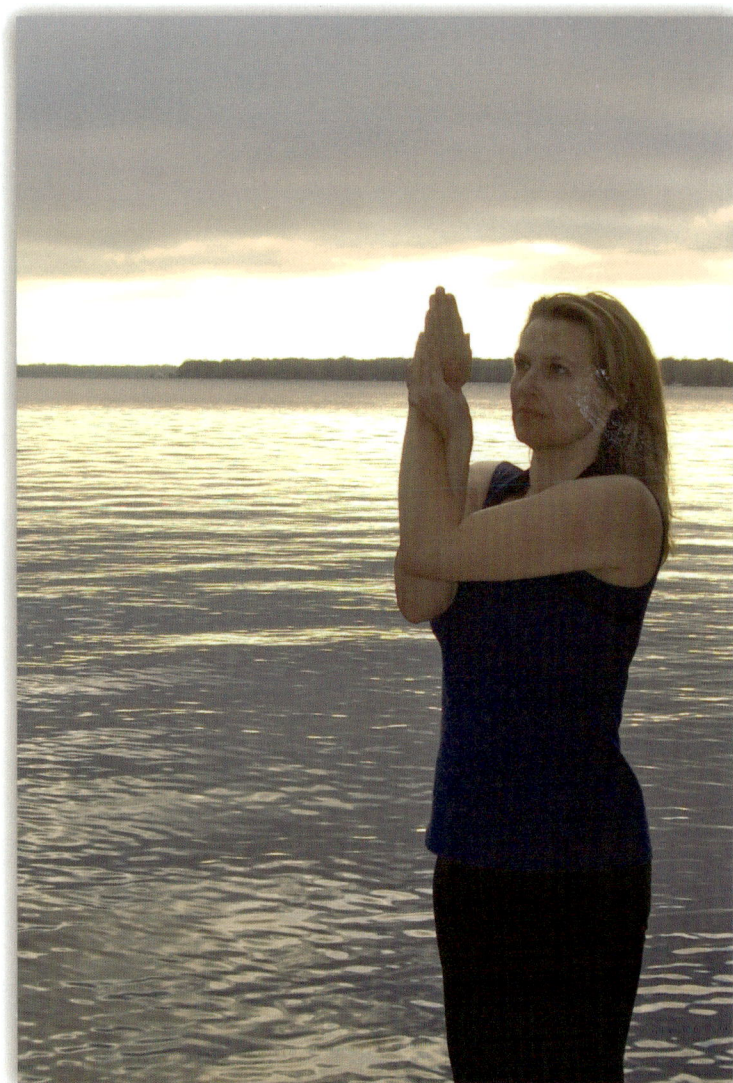

A TEA BATH FIT FOR A YOGINI

Do yourself a favor, pick up some bouquet garni sachets next time your in the market. Not only can you use them for a quickie soothing tonic like a bath tea but you can use them in your kitchen as well. The wonder of these little sachets is that they are reusable. Just clean and reuse again and again. There are two ways that I love to use these gems for my bath time rituals - you can simply toss one in and allow to steep, or you can tie it up under the hot faucet before filling the tub.

These herbs will work well in dried form. Simply crush or ground with your mortar and pestle.

3 tablespoons sea salt
1 tablespoon fennel
4 sprigs of lavender
4 tablespoons chamomile

Place all freshly ground ingredients into your bouquet garni sachet bag. To enjoy your bath tea, steep for a good 10 minutes.

YOGINI INSPIRED HAIR RINSE TONIC

This quick, homemade beauty trick will remove buildup from hair products and soften. Find beauty rituals like this one to add to your lifestyle. Compassionate, non-animal tested, homemade products are fun, cost effective, and leave you glowing.

1 ounce organic apple cider vinegar
1 quart spring water
1 hot towel

In a serving pitcher, combine the apple cider vinegar with the water and stir well. Pour over hair and wrap in hot towel for about 5 minutes. Rinse with warm to hot water.

Musing No. 67
The "imperfections" of her body adds character; her scars… add strength.

Didier Razon, E-RYT 500 hour, hails from St. Augustine, Florida and has been interested in yoga and the mystical side of life since his teenage years. On his own, he started practicing yoga asanas in Casablanca, Morocco, where he grew up. This was during the decade of the seventies where very few were familiar with this practice, let alone in Morocco! He received guidance in this endeavor by way of a couple of books in French by renowned yoga teacher Andre Van Lysbeth, who followed the Sivananda method.

In the early eighties, Didier traveled to India and Asia. In 1985, he had the great good fortune to meet Gurumayi Chidvilasananda in Ganeshpuri, India. Subsequently, due to this auspicious event, he spent the next ten years living in her ashrams (monasteries) in India, France, and the United States.

While living in the ashram, Didier had the opportunity to study hatha yoga with several teachers, notably John Friend - the founder of Anusara Yoga. Didier was, at one time, an Anusara affiliated teacher. He is presently certified through the Sivananda and Sri Mahesh Schools of Yoga.

In 2000, Didier created his own yoga school he named "Two Suns Rising Yoga." More information on Didier and his yogic life can be found at **www.didieryoga.com**. Rumi, a great Sufi poet saint (1207 - 1273) wrote a beautiful poem which alludes to this same theme that Didier lives his life, and it reads…

What a day today. There are two Suns rising! What a day, Not like any other day. Look! The Light is shining in your heart, The wheel of Life has stopped. Oh, you who can see into your own heart, What a day, This is your day. ~ Rumi

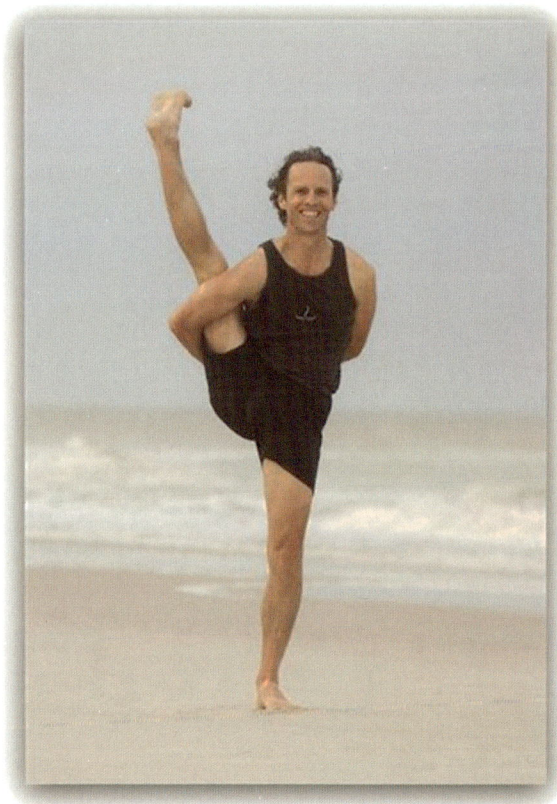

SWEET & SPICY YOGI TEA
serves 6-8

2 teaspoons ginger, freshly grated
3 cardamom seeds, bruised in mortar with pestle
6 - 8 whole cloves
1 teaspoon nutmeg, freshly grated
1 cinnamon stick
8 cups water
3 tablespoons rice milk
½ tablespoon agave nectar

In a medium saucepan add ginger, cardamom seeds, cloves, nutmeg, and cinnamon stick to water. Heat spiced mixture over medium-high heat for about 5 minutes. Strain into tea cup and add milk and agave nectar.

SHAMAN'S MINT TEA
serves 1

3 heaping tablespoons loose-leaf yerba maté
freshly grated nutmeg
2 cups spring water, hot
1 big sprig of fresh mint
1 tablespoon almond milk
½ tablespoon agave nectar

Pour yerba maté into press pot and generously grate nutmeg overtop the maté.

Fill French press pot with hot spring water, never boiling. Steep 5 minutes and plunge.

Don't brew longer than 5 minutes since maté becomes bitter with over-steeping. The French press method is ideal if you want to add other herbs or spices for additional flavor and benefits, not to mention no electricity is needed.

Choose one of your favorite cups and drop a large mint sprig in it. Pour hot maté over top.

Add almond milk and agave.

Andrew Misle hails from Edmonton, Canada. He grew up in Chile as the son of a famous Chilean entertainer, so it was natural for him to follow along. Moving to Canada at the age of 13 was challenging due to a language barrier. He found refuge in a multiple of disciplines. At 18 he became a certified Kung Fu instructor and in university, he was a member of the Bears wrestling team. His entertaining spirit pulled him into starring roles in both sitcoms and films. As a singer, Andrew toured alongside major acts and recorded three albums with a former band.

He has had a blast thus far, but the pursuit and achievement of personal goals came at a price. He found that the pursuit of his ambitions created a combination of stress and spiritual emptiness. Andrew found himself living his dreams without ever being quite present during the quest. Something had to change, so he stepped off the stage in search of deeper fulfillment and meaning.

"It's hard to tell whether I picked yoga or it picked me, and how I ended up in India studying it remains a mystery, but I do remember falling in love with yoga after my first Moksha class. The things Moksha stands for both inside and outside of the heated room are both humbling and inspirational. I feel incredibly blessed to be embraced by such a caring community. I'm grateful to yoga, I'm grateful to the great masters that came before me, I'm grateful to my teachers, and I'm grateful to life. I look forward to continuing to travel this path and passing on whatever jewels I gather along the way."

He spends his days currently teaching yoga full time on Prince Edward Island, while fulfilling a duality Sadhana through meditation, devoted study, and practice allowing theory to become practice and practice become theory.

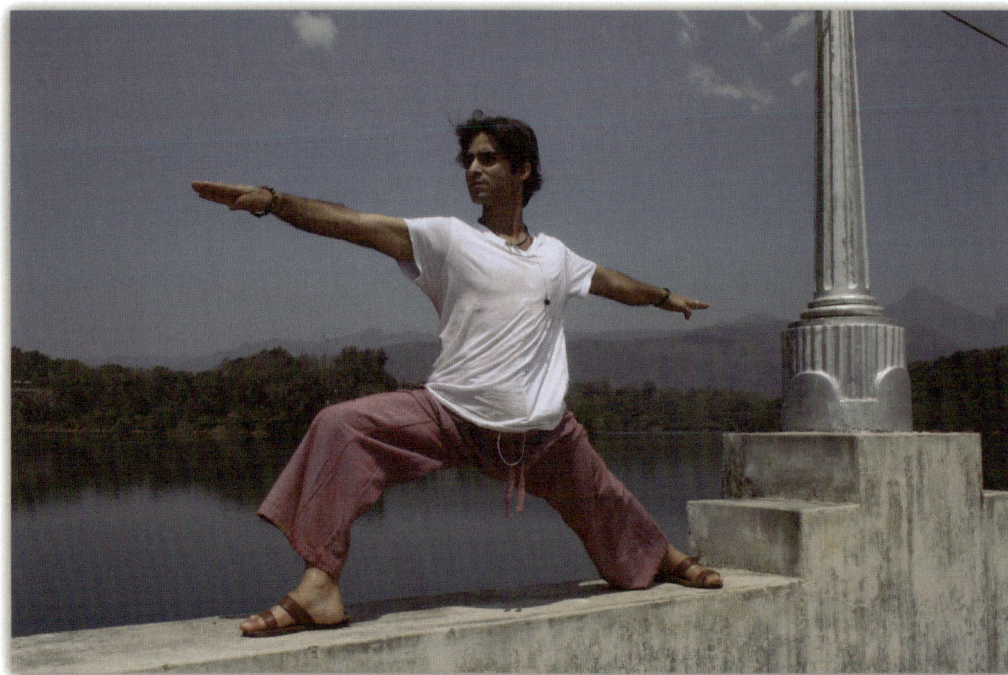

SHANTI SHAVING CREAM

4 tablespoons essential almond oil
2 tablespoons shea butter
1 ¾ cups distilled water
1 teaspoon baking soda
4 tablespoons castile soap, liquid (I like Dr. Bronner's)
¼ cup aloe vera gel
3 - 4 drops essential oil of pine

In a medium saucepan, heat the oil and shea butter in a double broiler. Stir consistently until mixture is clear. Pour mixture into a large bowl and set aside to cool.

In a separate pan, heat water, add in baking soda and soap, mix well. Add in the aloe vera gel and stir until thoroughly mixed. Pour soap and baking soda mixture into the bowl of oil and shea butter. Add in essential oil. With a hand mixer, blend all ingredients together for about 3 minutes. For best results blend a second time for about 2 - 3 minutes.

Store shaving cream in sterilized container in a cool, dry place. This has a shelf life of about 2 months.

Musing No. 68

You can be any religion to practice yoga, or none at all. Yoga is for all to use. Practice for clarity, for health, or for an overall state of tranquility.

Kishan Shah hails from Santa Monica, California and describes himself as "on the 21st Century Green Coalition, an abundant giant of expansive light, a warrior for peace, urban yogi, a storm chaser, jungle monkey, soul surfer, alchemistic shaman, mountain rider, and paradise seeker…a straight love junkie."

As a global teacher of Vinyasa Yoga and meditation, he leads workshops, retreats, and trains in some of the most beautiful places on planet earth. These teachings take a traditional standing on yoga, but Kishan then applies his 21st century life experiences like an alchemist developing a divine recipe for fields of unified consciousness. He combines dynamic recipes of Yoga Asana sequencing in sync with rhythmic breath patterns. His bottom line is, "inhale, and God remains with you. Exhale, and you approach God. Hold the exhalation, and surrender to God." (Krishnamacharya)

He is a practitioner of Ayurvedic Holistic Medicine. Ayurveda is the way to lead life balanced inline with the rhythms of nature. As yoga teaches us to breathe and prostrate, Ayurveda teaches us to eat and live. Kishan is currently finishing his clinical doctorate degree in Ayurveda after six years of study.

As a lecturer and an adjunct professor at UCLA in the World Arts and Cultures department, he has had the opportunity to lead hundreds of students through the practices of Vinyasa yoga, meditation, and Kalaripayyat movements. He also offers pure lecture based courses in the yoga philosophies of Samkhya philosophy and yoga sutras of Patanjali.

**Out beyond ideas of wrong doing and right doing, there is a field. I will meet you there.
~ Rumi**

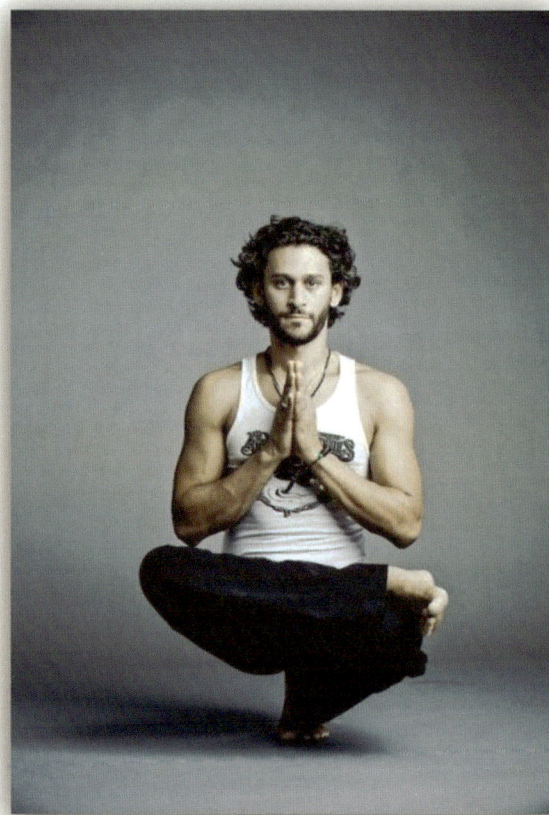

THE POST POWER YOGA SOAK

5 cups water
3 - 4 tablespoons ginger, freshly grated
1 cup Epsom salts

In a small sauce pan, heat water over medium-high heat. Put grated ginger in and cook for about 10 minutes. Remove ginger from water.

Pour salts in bath water, while water is running. Add gingered water mixture to the bath of warm salt water and soak for about 30 minutes.

BASIC CIDER TONICS
serves 1

Apple cider vinegar has a plethora of health benefits. This basic apple cider vinegar tonic recipe can help you with weight loss and boost energy when you are feeling fatigued. This will be a smidge on the bitter side, but think of the cleansing effects it will have on your body.

1 – 2 teaspoons organic apple cider vinegar
1 glass full glass of spring water

Mix apple cider vinegar in a glass of water. Take 3 times daily, before or during meals.

A warm cider tonic is wonderful as well.

1 - 2 teaspoons organic apple cider vinegar
1 cup hot water
2 teaspoons lime juice
2 teaspoons agave nectar

Stir all ingredients well.

Isaac Pena hails from New York City, NY and is the co-owner of Sankalpah Yoga. He began practicing martial arts at the age of seven and was introduced to Zen meditation at the age of nine. Zen meditation was his first experience with something deeper than the physical body. He began his yoga practice in the mid-nineties, taking daily classes from a wide variety of teachers.

In his desire to continue his education in Thai Body work, Isaac has made several trips to Thailand since 2000. He has received certification to practice Thai Body work and also to instruct others in the art under the guidance of Chung Kal and Chaiyuth Priyasith. In continuing to expand his knowledge of the body's potential, he has trained for several years in Contortion with Jonathan Nosan and personally trains other contortionist and circus performers. Through his experiences as a body worker, he is more able to meet people at their level and take them beyond their previous level of conditioning

It's an offering, deep from my heart. If it were just exercise or people moving mechanically, I couldn't do it. The chance that someone… hopefully everyone, will find in themselves is what makes my life so happy everyday. ~ Isaac Pena

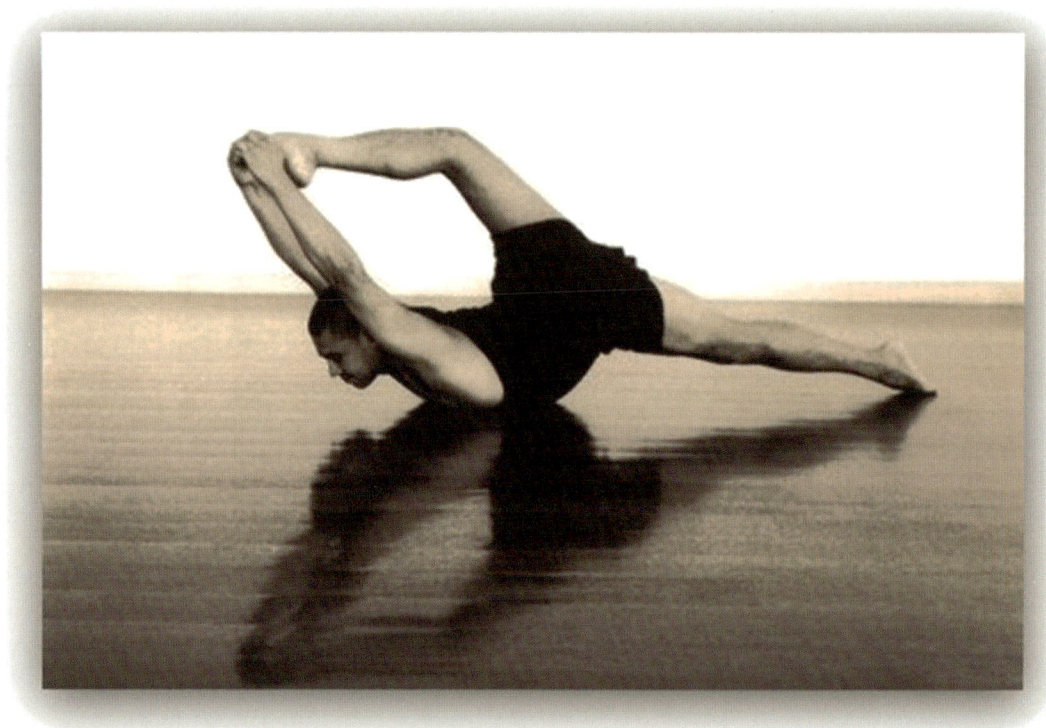

133

YOGI SWEET BARS
makes 15 bars

⅓ cup apricots, dried and chopped
⅓ cup medjool dates, chopped
¾ cup oat flour
⅓ cup raisins
1 cup sunflower seeds
3 bananas, mashed
1 ½ cups raw cane sugar
¾ teaspoon baking powder, aluminum free
¼ teaspoon sea salt

Preheat oven to 350 °F.

Oil a 10 x 10 baking dish with coconut oil. In a mixing bowl add apricots, dates, and 1 tablespoon of flour. Add in the raisins and seeds and set aside.

Place bananas and sugar in a medium mixing bowl and with a hand mixer, whip until mixture is blended, about 1 - 2 minutes.

Combine the remaining flour, baking powder, and salt in a separate bowl and fold in the banana mixture. Fold in the fruit and nut mixture.

Spread batter into the pre-oiled pan and bake until golden brown, about 20 minutes. Refrigerate for about an hour. Cut into bars.

A PRE-MEDITATION BASIL RUB

The aroma of basil is said to increase mental focus.

Soak basil in warm water for about 5 minutes, then dab on forehead, wrists, and under nose before meditation.

Penny Powell RYT, 200 hour, hails from Jacksonville, Florida is a juice enthusiast, yoga teacher, and creator of JuicYoga™. As a mother, wife, and friend, Penny has found ways to incorporate doses of nutrition and centeredness in her home and community.

"Maybe it's because the practices of juicing and yoga nourish the body at the cellular level that I feel so alive when partaking of them. I truly FEEL something from juicing and yoga! After drinking a freshly-made juice, I almost instantly feel healthier, more alive, and more connected to my soul and my surroundings. My gratitude for life increases, and I often find myself standing in awe of nature's beauty and bounty. Even simply handling produce in preparation for the juicer does something positive for my well-being. Then, when pushing the colorful fruits and veggies through the juicer, I marvel at how the produce so beautifully transforms to a liquid loaded with nutrients that virtually becomes instant nutrition for the body due to the little-to-no-digestion process that juices require.

SIPPING ON SUNSHINE

Inspired by the solar plexus chakra
A tropical infused concoction

Feed all ingredients through the juicer. Feel free to adjust the quantities to your needs. Juice, stir, and add ice if would like your juice on the rocks.

2 - 3 inch slices pineapple, peeled
2 star fruits
3 - 4 yellow apples
1 thumb tip ginger

The spicy kick that the ginger root offers will provide you with a wide range of benefits. Ginger can help calm stomach issues, relieve arthritis, and help fight off colds. Add this spicy root to boost many dishes, or add it to some sunshine and stars for a luminous, bright juice!

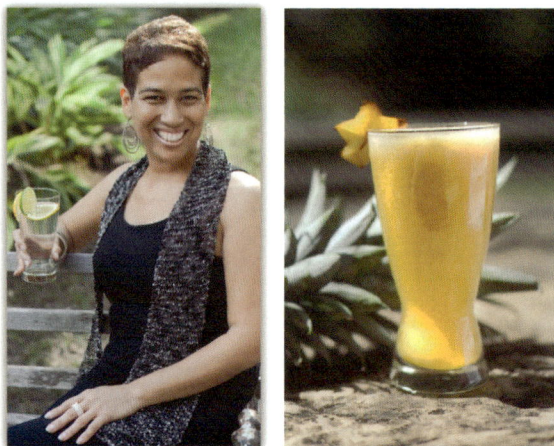

Chloe Longobardo-Moreno hails from Queens, New York and is wife to her beloved, Elias Moreno. Chloe is a step-mom, eBay entrepreneur, TNR certified, Army Veteran, and lover of all souls and nature. She has followed a love of the Arts via studying at a university in Commercial Art, Jewelry Design, and a field study of Modern Arts in Paris. Chloe is an inspiration to her family and many friends…her smile and zest for a healthy lifestyle has inspired others to try new options in the kitchen. Chloe's personality can be summed up with her favorite quote…."Don't panic, go organic!". Her enthusiasm of holistic, ethical, and overall health and wellbeing has given her life a complete balance.

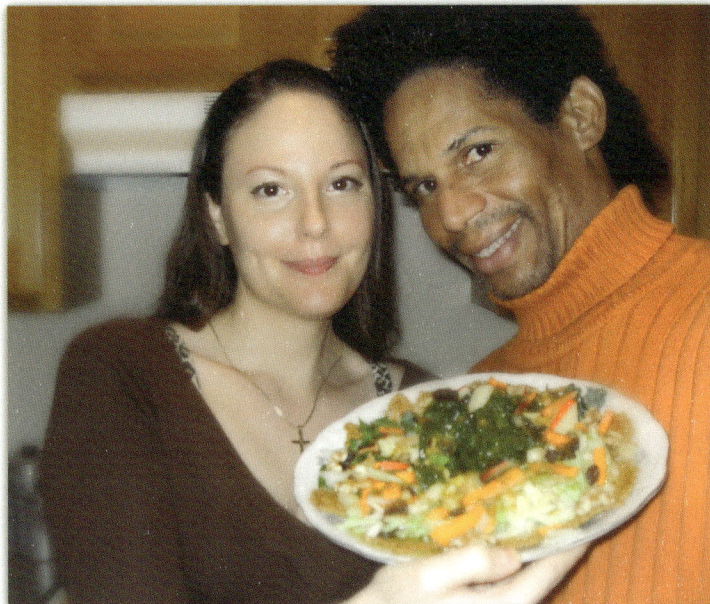

GREENS TO THE MAX WITH FLAX SALAD

serves 2

1 handful of dandelion greens
1 bunch bock choy (leaves)
¼ of small green cabbage
1 handful Lacinato kale
several cloves raw garlic, chopped (we used probably 10 or more)
⅓ of a large yellow onion, chopped
a couple of shallots, chopped
1 big carrot, chop into small pieces
½ cup walnuts, chop into small pieces
½ cup raisins
sprouted sunflower seeds (sprinkle small handful on top)
flax crackers (Foods Alive Mexican Harvest; take several crackers & break into smaller pieces)
½ of an apple, chopped into small pieces
4 tablespoons Bragg's Apple Cider Vinegar
4 tablespoons extra virgin olive oil
4 tablespoons maple syrup
Trocomare herb seasoning (sprinkle on; adjust to taste)
cayenne (sprinkle on; adjust to taste)
turmeric (sprinkle on; adjust to taste)

Mix all ingredients well. Enjoy!

Mitzi Mager hails from Pennsylvania and is a wife, mother of three (Hailey, Sydney, and Alek), entrepreneur, and fierce advocate for those who do not have a voice. **"Vegan for the animals and environment first, for health second…every living being deserves the chance to live in peace."**
She is a metal smith and jewelry designer by trade being drawn to uniquely expressing the timeless beauty of nature through artistic mediums of gemstones, glass, and precious metals. Her custom craft is inspired by nature and all her wonderful colors; her compassion designs tailored alterations for special needs. She accomplishes all this, and yet takes the time to find the humor in life, "laughing so hard tears roll down your face and you can't breath!"

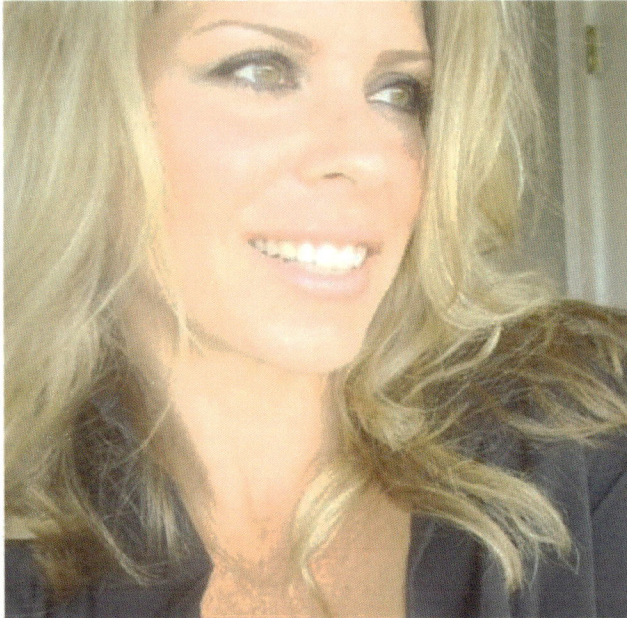

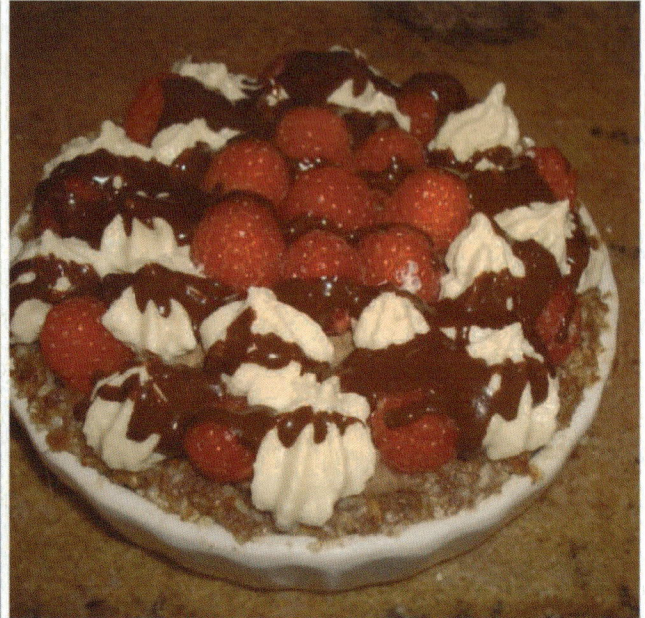

CHOCOLATE CREAM PIE
serves 6 - 8

CRUST

1 cup raw almonds
1 cup raw pecans
1 - 2 teaspoons cinnamon
½ teaspoon Celtic salt
2 tablespoons cacao powder
2 tablespoons coconut oil/butter
2 teaspoons alcohol free vanilla
9 dates, pitted and finely chopped (soaking them is optional)
6 tablespoons coconut shavings
2 - 3 tablespoons raw agave nectar

Place all ingredients into a food processor and pulse until crust consistency is reached. Press crust into pan, pie plate, or tart pans.

FILLING

2 ½ cups soaked raw cashews (soak for at least 3 hours)
4 teaspoons alcohol free vanilla extract
1 ½ cups cacao powder
⅓ cup coconut water
1 - 2 ½ cups almond milk
¼ cup raw agave nectar
⅓ cup coconut oil
1 Haas avocado
1 teaspoon chocolate extract (optional)

Blend raw cashews with the vanilla, coconut water, almond milk, and chocolate extract (optional) in the food processor. Move to blender and add remaining ingredients. This is the part where your own taste will dictate the ingredient's measurements. I find the adjustments to be mainly based on the cacao and agave.

Keep scraping sides of blender and pushing down to get a very thorough blending!

WHIPPED "CREAM"

1 cup soaked cashews (soaked for at least 3 hours)
½ cup almond milk
1 teaspoon pure vanilla extract
1 tablespoon raw agave nectar
1 teaspoon lemon juice from fresh lemon
1 tablespoon coconut oil

Blend all ingredients until smooth and fluffy. Be sure to scrape sides of blender and push everything down to reach the blades.

Musing No. 69

Nibble on fresh edamame, blueberries, or cherries picked that day or fresh from the Farmers' Market! There's no doubt that these add a rather nutrient-rich layer of goodness to a scrumptious sandwich or when simply eaten alone.

Ayinde Howell hails from New York City, NY and is an entrepreneur, executive vegan chef, actor, musician, writer, and founder of **www.ieatgrass.com.** Howell, born in a small town called Tacoma, Washington, is a lifelong vegan who started practicing yoga with his family at the age of ten. He has a background in a variety of vegan fare covering soul food, raw, and new American. He is a freelance executive Vegan Chef. His most recent position was a two year post as executive chef of the JivamkTea Café in Union Square, NYC. He is also founder of and co-owner of Hillside Quickie's Vegan Sandwich Shop, an offshoot of the family business. HQVSS became a popular lunch spot known for blasting hip hop during the crowded rushes and being frequented by notable industry clients like The Roots, Saul Williams, Common, Blackalicious, and the Erykah Badu when their respective tours came through town. **He is currently working on his first cookbook** *I Eat Grass, A Lifestyle Book.*

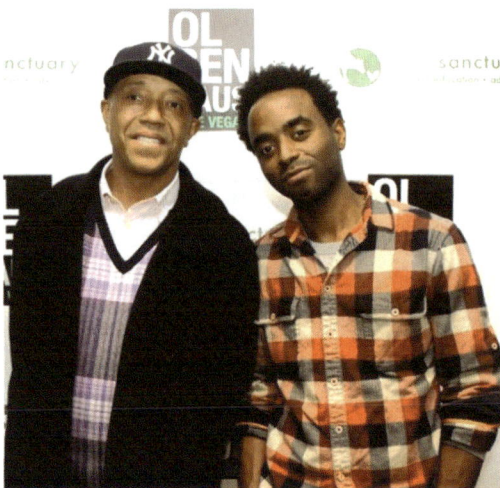

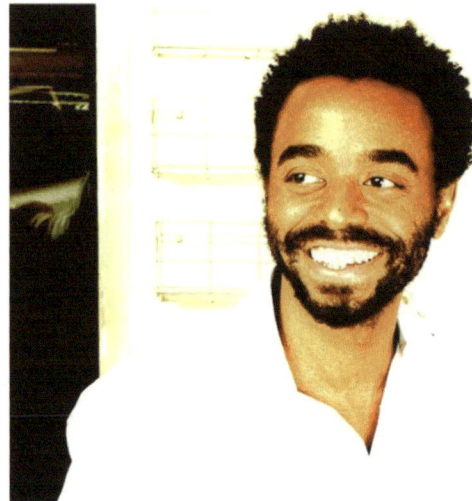

BEER BATTERED TEMPEH TACOS

1 pound tempeh (sliced in strips)
½ cup canola, safflower, or corn oil
2 cups white cabbage (shredded)
1 small onion (sliced)

MARINADE

1 ½ cups soy sauce
½ cup vinegar
1 tablespoon dry basil
1 tablespoon dry oregano
1 tablespoon chili powder
1 teaspoon dry thyme
1 stick kombu

WHITE SAUCE

1/2 cup vegan plain yogurt
1/2 cup vegan sour cream
1 lime, juiced
1 jalapeno or habenero pepper, seeded minced
1/2 teaspoon ground cumin
1 tablespoon fresh dill weed
1 teaspoon crushed red pepper

BATTER

1 cup all purpose flour
2 tablespoons cornstarch
1 teaspoon baking powder, aluminum free
½ teaspoon salt
½ teaspoon black pepper
1 ½ cups beer (I use ale)
1 ½ teaspoon Ener-g egg replacer
3 tablespoons warm water

METHOD:

1. Marinade: Mix soy sauce and vinegar in mixing bowl. Add basil, oregano, chili, thyme and kombu. Mix well. Add tempeh and cover, allowing to marinade for 40 minutes.

2. In a separate bowl, add mayo and yoghurt mix. Add lime juice until sauce is runny. Mix in herbs and jalapeno and taste. it should have a spicy, limey dill flavor.

*Preheat a medium sauce pot with oil over a medium high flame. Warm tortillas wrapped in foil in over at 350°F.

3. Mix flour, cornstarch, baking powder, salt, and black pepper in a separate bowl. In a small bowl, whip up Ener-g egg replacer with water until frothy. Add beer and quickly add to dry mix mixing with your whisk. A few lumps are ok. Remove tempeh from marinade, dust with remaining flour dip and cover in batter. Drop into hot oil. Tempeh will float to the top, turn with tongs. Cook until golden brown on both sides.

4. Fill warm tortillas with two pieces of tempeh, a handful of shredded white cabbage, some raw onion, and white sauce.

Drew McCall Burke hails from South County, Rhode Island and is mom to three beautiful children and wife for 23 years. She is a professional fitness trainer, certified in spinning, yoga, and Pilates. She holds a degree in Physical Therapy specializing in sports rehabilitation. In the juicing community, she is known as "The Juice Babe." She is a co-author of a screenplay called "Nature's Law" and creator of Sexy Raw Vegan 5 Day Juicy Fast program. It is available at VEGANREALITY.COM so that you can…loose weight, feel great, and get your sexy on! Detox and cleanse your way to an uber, lean, and sexy earthling.

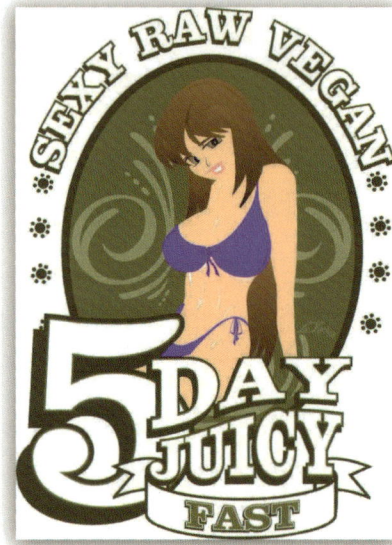

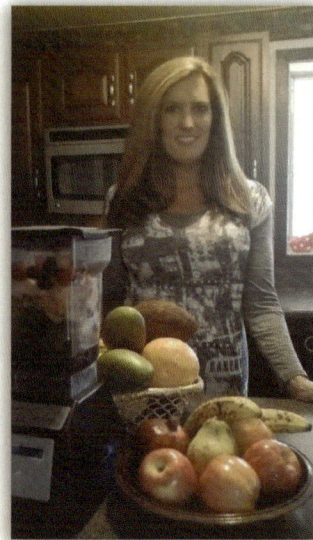

TROPICAL SALAD WITH TZAZIKI DRESSING

1 head romaine lettuce
2 sliced cucumbers
2 cans mandarin oranges, drained
2 sliced avocadoes
2 sliced mangos

In a large bowl, mix lettuce, cucumbers, mandarin oranges, avocadoes, mangos. Make dressing.

TZAZIKI DRESSING

juice of two limes
½ chopped cilantro
1 chopped jalapeño
½ cup chopped mint
2 chopped cucumbers, no seeds or skin
1 clove of chopped garlic
5 - 8 ounces of coconut yogurt

Chop cucumber, and drain off excess liquid.

In a medium bowl combine, lime juice, cilantra, jalapeno, mint, cucumber, and garlic. Chop all ingredients into tiny pieces before adding to coconut yogurt.

Let chill in fridge for at least 2 hours. Pour Tzaziki Dressing over salad and serve.

Oli Dillon Squire hails from Ludlow, United Kingdom, Oli is blazing a trail of advocacy for those who cannot speak for themselves, creating a tsunami against corruption in government and the unspeakably, horrific acts against Mother and her children. His website **www.actionforourplanet.com** highlights his current actions including the fight against the fur industry. He has garnered world wide notability and respect which is shown in the responses from both individuals and corporations such as numerous celebrities, Cartier luxury watch manufacturer, and the fashion industry. As busy as Oli stays, he has shared one of his favorite dishes he enjoys preparing.

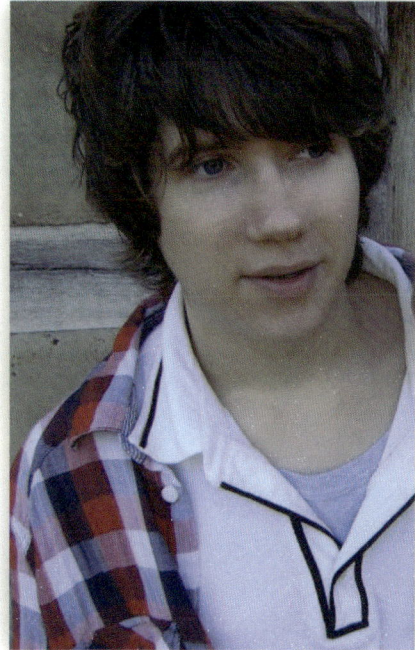

A LUDLOW DINNER
serves 4

4 red peppers, tops precut and seeded
extra virgin olive oil
1 12 oz packet organic tempeh, cut into strips
1 red onion diced
½ cup of sliced mushrooms
2 teaspoons dried oregano
3 tablespoons Braggs
1 16 ounce tin of tomato puree
1 16 ounce tin of diced tomatoes
2 bay leaves
fresh chopped parsley (optional)

Preheat oven to 375 °F

Use oven-proof dish with oil, and cook peppers for approximately 20 minutes

Then, using a wok, add olive oil, and cook the tempeh over medium high heat. Cook tempeh until golden brown on both sides. Add onion, mushrooms, and oregano.

Cook for 10 minutes, stirring regularly. Add tomato puree, tin of tomatoes, and bay leaves. Add a small amount of cold water; cook for another 10 minutes.

Fill the cooked peppers with mixture, and garnish with parsley. It's now ready to serve and can be served with a whole wheat pasta, or brown rice. I like to sprinkle mine with a soy cheddar cheese.

Ron Prasad hails from Melbourne, Victoria, Australia and is a steadfast animal activist who embraces a vegan lifestyle for the ethics and compassion it gives all life. He is the author of the self-help book *Welcome to Your Life*.

He became vegetarian at age 17, journeying into a vegan at age 31. Early in life he knew his mission was being a relentless advocate for animal rights and to help rekindle a sense of self-worth and compassion within people. Involved in a number of groups, he has done work for some of Australia's most well known animal rights organizations and shelters. He enjoys playing the guitar to resonate with the rhythm in his mind and loves to be a 'daddy' to his German Shepherd, Kefu, who warms his heart and soul.

THE AUSSIE CAKE
serves 6 - 8

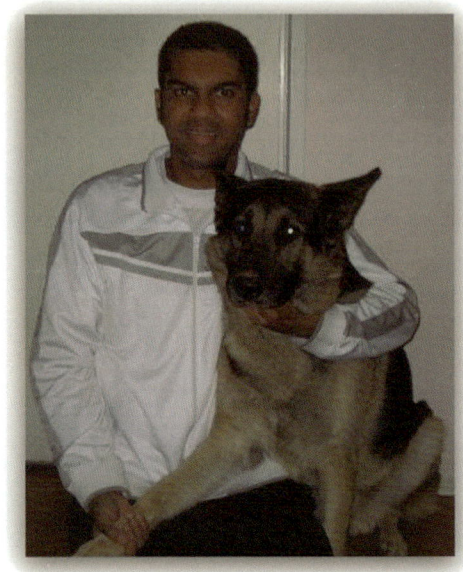

As Ron is an Aussie…the measurements below will need to be converted as needed.

300 grams of whole meal self-rising flour
100 grams raw brown sugar
200 grams desiccated coconut (grated, dried coconut)
2 tablespoons of raw organic cocoa powder
200 ml coconut oil
200 ml of water
2 medium sized ripe bananas, mashed
2 portions of "Egg Replacer" (as per instructions on the packet)

Preheat oven to 160 °C. Oil and flour pan.

In a large bowl mix flour, sugar, coconut, and cocoa. In a separate bowl mix oil, water, bananas, and Egg Replacer. Slowly beat the dry ingredients into the wet ingredients. Pour mixture into pan.

Bake for 45 minutes. Allow cake cool and serve.

Tracy Shearer hails from a small town in Pennsylvania just outside of Philadelphia where she lives with her family. She has forged a personal path by detail documenting her ups and downs of her lifestyle transformation from omnivore to vegan. She is truly finding she is happy being a free spirit and living her yoga. She has encountered many *Om Mani Pad Me Hum* moments (a mantra meaning "generosity, ethics, patience, diligence, renunciation, and wisdom"). By having the forethought to create brutally honest observations of this quest, she is providing a space of empathy and information. She offers a refuge for anyone who needs encouragement and comfort from an unhealthy and resentful world. Tracy explains her "circle of safety" and how this benefits her in a co-existence with the extremely negative reactions from non-vegans in everyday life.

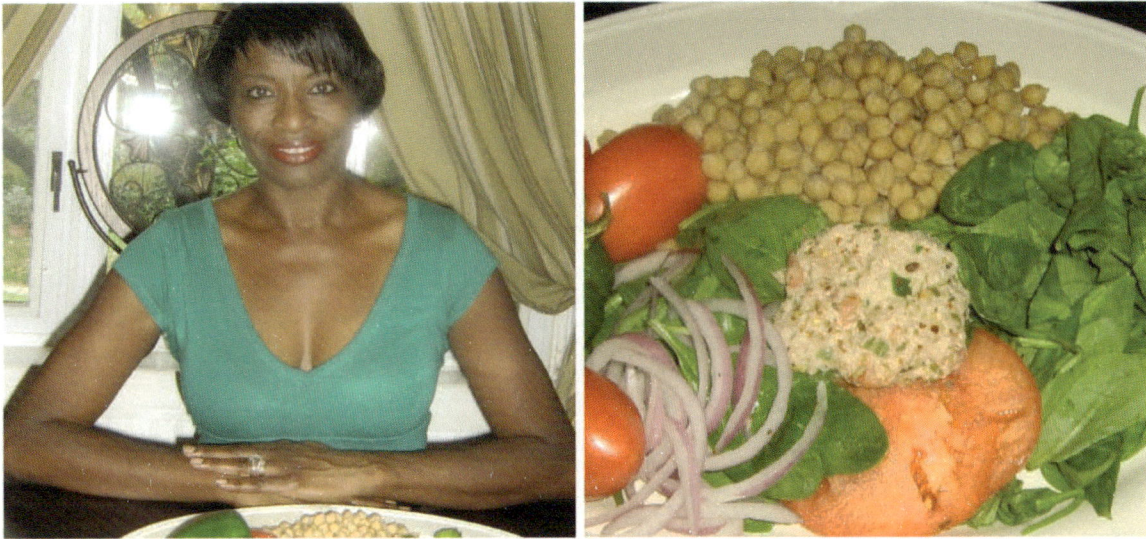

VEGGIE TUNA
serves 2

1 cup chick peas (garbanzo beans), cooked and ground
½ cup red onions, diced
½ tomato, diced
½ green pepper, diced
2 cloves fresh garlic, finely diced
½ teaspoon crushed red, hot pepper flakes
sea salt and fresh ground pepper to taste
2 tablespoons vegan mayonnaise

In a medium bowl, mix chick peas, onion, tomato, green pepper, and garlic. Fold in hot pepper flakes, salt, ground pepper and mayo. Serve and enjoy!

Ursula Zamora Ursula Zamora hails from Pinellas Park, Florida where she lives with her family, but her hometown is Williamson, NY. Although her career as a Freelance Media and PR Facebook Administrator keeps her very busy, she makes time to use natural remedies for her family's health and well-being. Her creative and intuitive approaches to healthful tonics and tasty meals brings her family joy. She is a beacon of inspiration to all mothers she meets and happy to spread encouragement with her knowledge of a holistic lifestyle.

VEGGIE MISH-MASH SAUTÉ

A favorite meatless meal for me is putting any number of veggies together, but this is our family favorite.

1 tablespoon coconut or olive oil
one large onion, halved then sliced
½ each: green, red, and yellow peppers,
    (sliced lengthwise)
1 large Portobello mushroom, halved and sliced
3 or 4 large tomatoes, seeded and diced
a handful of collard leaves; stemmed, halved and
cut into "chunks" (you can use baby spinach if you do
not like collards)
2 large garlic cloves, peeled and thinly sliced
handful of fresh basil leaves, cut chiffonade-style or torn
1 zucchini, halved and chunked
sea salt and fresh ground pepper to taste

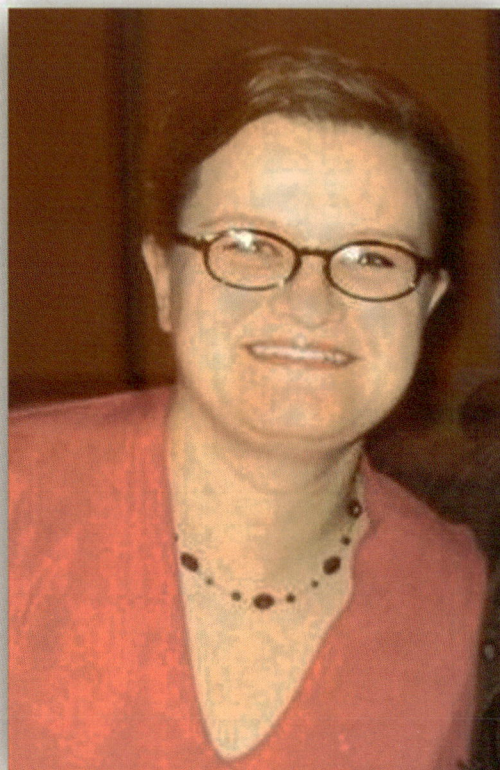

In a large pan or cast iron pot, add oil and onions. Sauté onions until transparent, and add peppers and Portobello. When peppers have cooked about halfway, add tomatoes. Cook the tomatoes down for about 10 minutes or so, and then add the collard greens. Cook them for another 5 minutes or so, and add the garlic, basil and zucchini (if you like, red wine, a dash of good red wine can be added here as well). Cook everything together for another 5 - 10 minutes, and then add salt and pepper to taste.

Jace Kai hails from New York, New York where he was born and raised. He works as a photographer and is a published poet, short story writer, and will be designing one of many video games. With all these artful endeavors, he still finds time for his true passion…animal rights. Many interests exude within Jace, tattoos, astronomy, mythology, and trips to Disney World. However, his trueness speaks in his love for the souls of the ones that do not have a voice. Jace Kai uses a strong voice full of gumption, moxie, and compassion. He is an un-movable force for the many souls that deserve to live a life without inhumane acts done against them.

URBAN INFUSED DINNER
serves 2

1 pound Tri-color vegetable pasta (carrot, tomato and spinach)
1 cup baby corn
1/2 cup water chestnuts
1 cup bean sprouts
1 cup bamboo shoots
1 carrot, sliced into thin strips
1/4 cup low sodium soy sauce
1/4 cup low sodium Teriyaki sauce
1 clove fresh garlic, peeled and minced
1 tablespoon olive oil
freshly ground black pepper to taste
dried red pepper to taste
1 tablespoon red chili sauce
1/4 cup juice of 1 freshly squeezed lime
1/2 cup grape tomatoes, chilled and sliced
fresh sprigs of dill, optional

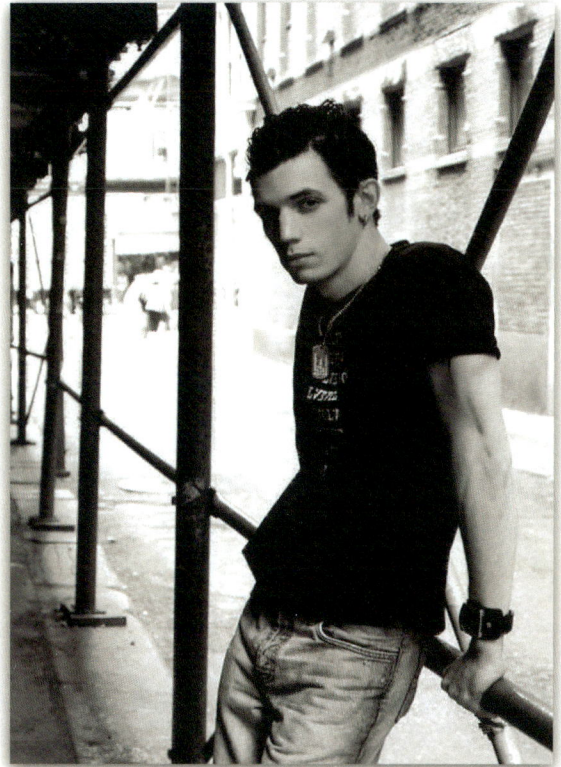

Marinate the baby corn, water chestnuts, bean sprouts, bamboo shoots, and carrot slices in the soy & teriyaki sauces. While the vegetables are marinating, prepare the remaining ingredients. Boil the pasta according to the directions, and drain. Toast the garlic pieces. Once cooked, arrange the pasta on a plate. Add the marinated vegetables on top. Drizzle the pasta mixture with garlic & olive oil. Finish with a few cold sliced mini tomatoes positioned on the side. Sprinkle the tomatoes with the toasted garlic pieces, olive oil, and garlic powder. Add salt, and black pepper to taste. Garnish with dill.

Zenita Belle hails from Champaign, Illinois with her husband and two rescue cats, Yoshi and Luna. The two are from the twin cities and home of the University of Illinois. She loves to travel especially to Colorado Springs in the summer, where nature seems to seep in and surround her with a divine energy. Creating and indulging in one of a kind vegan dishes has become not only a hobby but also a way of life for her and her family. One of her favorite recipes is offered to you to create and indulge in as well…enjoy!

TACOS WITH STUFFED POBLANO PEPPERS

serves 4

1 cup brown rice
1 teaspoon cumin
1 teaspoon smoked paprika
1 teaspoon garlic powder
1 teaspoon onion powder
sea salt and fresh ground pepper to taste
½ cup Daiya vegan shredded cheddar cheese
1 pint cherry tomatoes cut into quarters
1 15-oz. can of corn
4 large Poblano peppers, seeded and sliced up the middle, but not cut in half
1 15-oz. can of enchilada sauce (hot or mild)
1 10-count package of flat bottom corn taco shells
2 cups guacamole
1 ½ cups shredded romaine lettuce
1 15-oz. can of sliced black olives

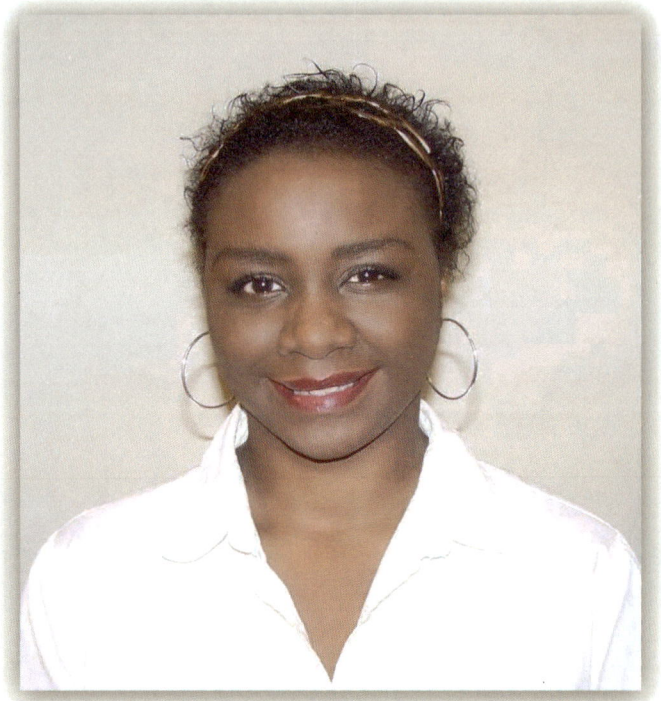

Preheat oven to 400 °F.

Cook rice according to package directions. Once rice is cooked, add cumin, paprika, garlic, onion, salt, pepper, Daiya cheese, tomatoes, and corn.

Spray an 8 ½ x 8 ½ baking pan with cooking spray (or wipe down with your favorite cooking oil).

With a tablespoon, take rice mixture and began to stuff peppers until full. Once all peppers are stuffed, place into pan and drizzle the enchilada sauce over them.

Place into oven. Cook for 40 minutes.

Prepare Bean & Salsa mixture.

Once peppers are done, take out of oven and let cool. Remove beans from heat.

Microwave taco shells for 25 seconds, and begin to assemble tacos. Take a taco shell and line bottom with a layer of guacamole, bean mixture, lettuce, tomatoes, sliced black olives, salsa, cilantro, and Daiya vegan cheese.

Plate tacos, and use a spatula to remove stuffed peppers from pan and add to plate.

Sprinkle plate with remaining cilantro and a few tomatoes. Serve and enjoy!

BEAN & SALSA MIXTURE

1 15-oz. can of pinto beans
1 15-oz. can of refried black beans with limejuice
1 15-oz. can of diced tomatoes with jalapeno's and green chilies
2 medium bunches of fresh cilantro
cooking spray

Open can of pinto beans, drain, and place into a medium sized pot, and mash roughly or pulse in a food processor until roughly chopped. Add refried black beans, and bring to a small boil over medium heat. Turn down to low and let simmer, stirring occasionally.

ENRIQUE RUIZ LECHON hails from, Cancun, Quintana Roo, Mexico. He is a die-hard surfer who loves the waves of the oceans of life and cherishes each moment. Enrique plays the guitar, works in real estate, travels, loves snorkeling and deep sea diving, an avid skate boarder, yoga enthusiast, and has been recently enjoying time swimming in the deep ocean with our beloved creatures of the sea…whales. Enjoying compassionate foods, hanging with friends and family is quite simply all that is required for a most amazing life experience for Enrique. Carpe Diem ~ It's not just the length of life, but it's the "waves" of life.

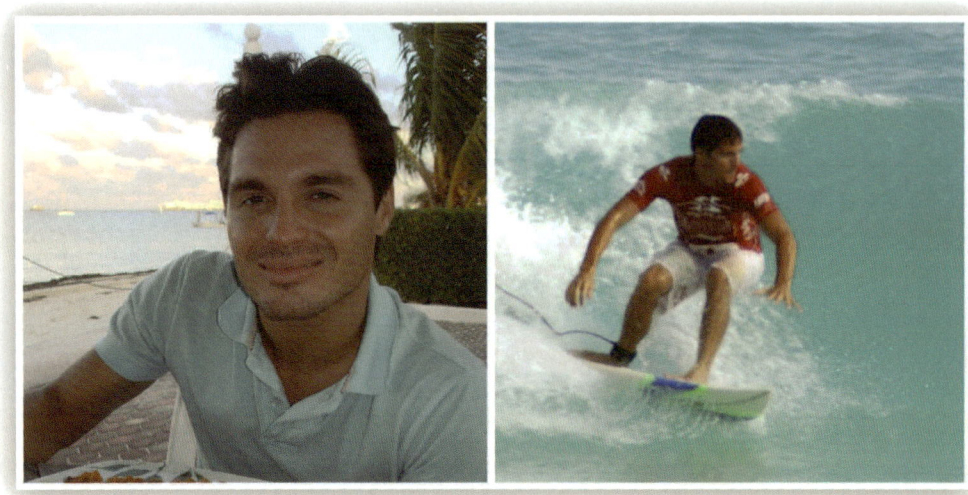

FENNEL LEMONY BOWL OF SOUL

serves 4

This simplistic yet soulful bowl of goodness is a must have in your stash of soups…indulge in the simple things in life…for the simple things are what makes for the most amazing life experience.

½ cup extra virgin olive oil
½ cup fresh squeezed lemon juice
2 cloves garlic, minced
5 cups vegetable broth
sea salt and fresh ground pepper to taste
1 fennel bulb, shaved and chopped
2 scallions, chopped

Blend oil, lemon juice, garlic, and veggie broth in blender until smooth. Season with salt and pepper to taste. Top each bowl with shaved fennel and scallions.

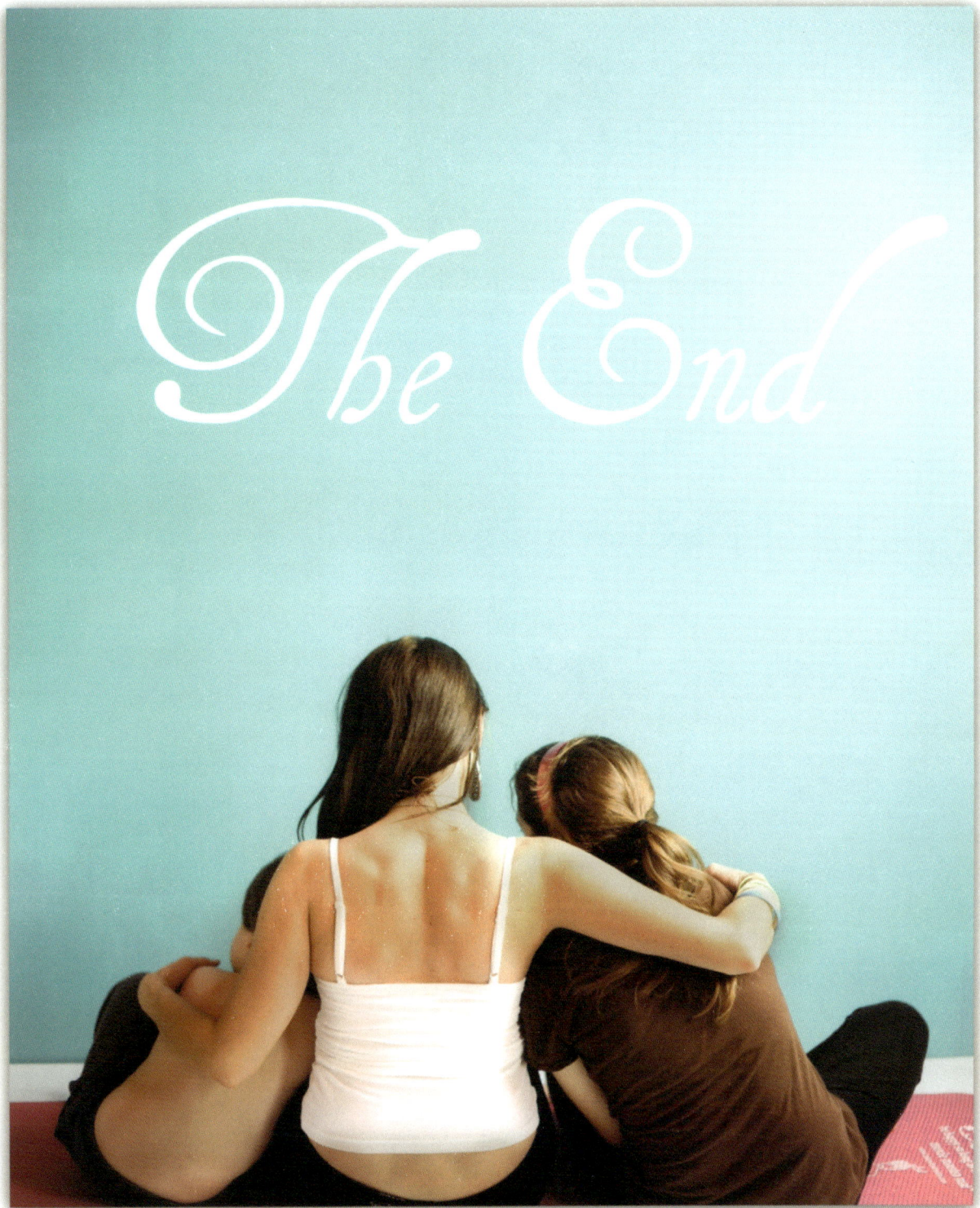

WE WISH YOU SHANTI AND LIGHT... FIND IT WITHIN YOURSELF, IT WILL BE THE GREATEST GIFT. WE WISH YOU MANY ENCHANTING MOMENTS... THE LITTLE THINGS IN LIFE, INSPIRED GATHERINGS... GIGGLES OF CHILDREN IN YOUR HOME! WE WISH YOU DAYS OF LIVING WARMLY FROM THE HEART AND NIGHTS FULL OF STARRY CELEBRATIONS. WE WISH YOU BLISSFUL SURPRISES.... THE ONES THAT LIFT YOUR SPIRIT, AND KISS YOUR SOUL FOREVER.   - CHARLIE, MADISON & JULES

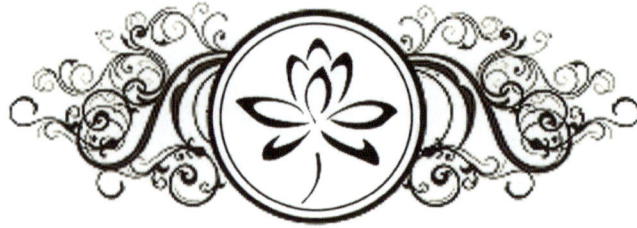

CREDITS

RUTH SHEPHERD

KRISTEN ASHTON

RENEE WEAVER

MICHAEL PHELAN

IAN KEOGH

ERIC LUSION

BE PRESENT

V UNITE

GARDEN OF LIFE

CHAKRAS BY DIDI

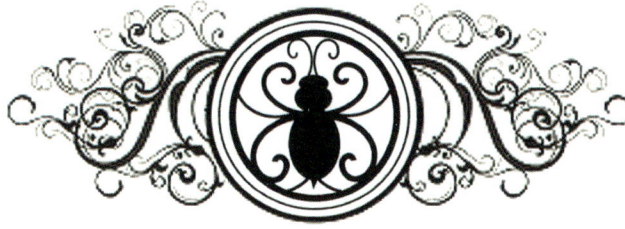

INDEX

A

B

U

V

W

Y

TOP FAVORITE WEBSITES

WWW.THEVEGANMUSE.COM

WWW.DIDIERYOGA.COM

WWW.GRACEOFTHEHEARTHEALING.COM

WWW.YOGAANANDASTUDIO.COM

WWW.NEWPARADIGMBOOK.COM

WWW.ACTIONFOROURPLANET.COM

WWW.SELINANATURALLY.COM

WWW.MOOPIGNATURALS.COM

WWW.MOOPIGVEGAN.COM

WWW.VEGANREALITY.COM

WWW.PETA.COM

WWW.YOGAGIRLGOESVEGAN2.BLOGSPOT.COM

WWW.THEGRASSROOTSMARKET.COM

LaVergne, TN USA
30 March 2011
222093LV00003B